Date Due

ᴅᴇᴄ 90

ROE-SHERIDAN LAKE LIBRARY

OCT 26 1991

FEB 28 1992

BEAUTY WORKS

HOW TO LOOK 10 YEARS YOUNGER

BEAUTY WORKS

HOW TO LOOK 10 YEARS YOUNGER

Arline Usden

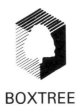

BOXTREE

First published in Great Britain in 1990
by Boxtree Limited

Designed by **Penny Mills**
Illustrated by **Lynne Robinson**
Photography (jacket, pp. 6 and 65–68): **Peter Underwood**
Hair by **Richard Dalton** at Claridges
Make-up by Vanessa Haines for **Max Factor**
Edited by **Margaret Adolphus**
Typeset by **York House Typographic**
Printed in England by **Clays Ltd, St Ives plc**

For Boxtree Limited
36 Tavistock Street
London
WC2E 7PB

British Library Cataloguing in Publication Data
Usden, Arline
   Beauty works: how to look ten years younger.
   1. Women.   Beauty care
   I. Title
   646.72082

ISBN 1-85283-286-X

CONTENTS

	INTRODUCTION	7
1	Save your skin	10
2	Laying foundations	34
3	All about eyes	42
4	Lip service	59
5	Taking steps	65
6	Arts & craftiness	69
7	A show of hands	72
8	On your feet	77
9	Neck's time	85
10	Beyond the fringe	91
11	Operation beauty	108
12	Beat the clock	120
	INDEX OF BEAUTY PROBLEMS	128
	USEFUL ADDRESSES	129
	PICTURE CREDITS	130

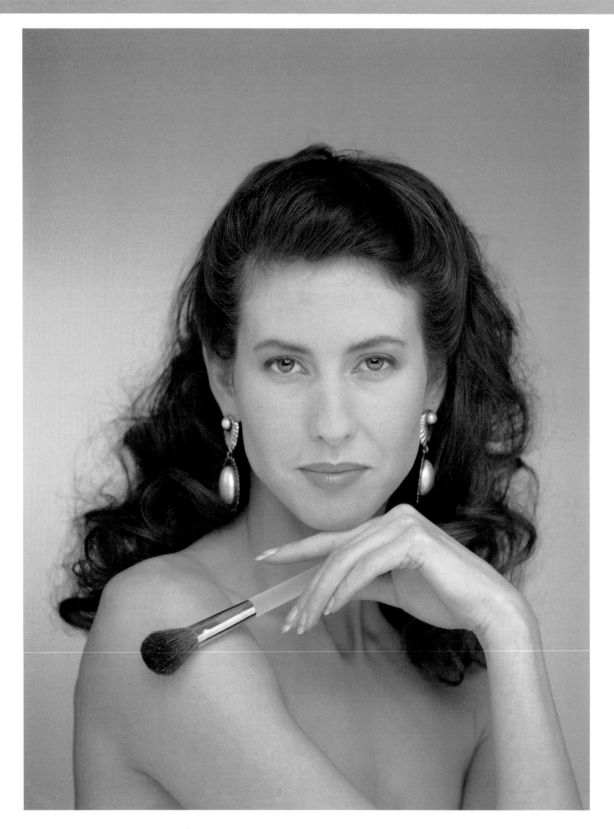

INTRODUCTION

We have been trying to stave off the wrinkles and hold back the inexorable onslaught of time and ageing since the Pharaohs and probably even before that, although as the lifespan was short, and you could be old at 30, there wasn't the impetus there is today.

The Victorian woman was old, nay ancient, by 40, but today being 40 is just a blip on the calendar, with 40-year-olds doing as much as ever they did at 23, and more determined than ever to stay young-looking as long as possible.

In fact, the 40s are today what the 30s were yesteryear, and the 50s are more like the 40s. Apple-cheeked old ladies may traditionally start around 70, but they're not so keen on the 'old' label either, thank you very much. We all want to look good and feel good for as long as we can because it improves the quality of our lives.

What Puritan could deny us that? What is there about age that we should want to give in gracefully? Personally I don't want to give in, at all, and I have a great admiration for those who manage to keep the old Reaper at bay with all the energy and skill that they can summon up.

That is not to say that we should be dressing like a 16-year-old at 46 or adopting a make-up and style that is distinctly and embarrassingly out of place. Feeling young and looking great, whatever your age, does not mean dressing and acting inappropriately, but is a combination of looks, mental stimulus, personality, confidence, health, fitness, vitality and motivation. And the one really good thing about getting older, experience, can be utilized in everything we attempt to do.

Of course, there have been many remedies for ageing, and lately, psychologists have been coming round to the view that it is love and sex that keeps you looking young. In a study of 700 youthful-looking over-40s, senior psychologist Dr David Weeks of the Edinburgh Hospital's Jardine Clinic, investigating scientific theories of ageing, discovered that half had partners on average 12 years younger.

'Most have always enjoyed a very vigorous sex life. They have a high sex drive and often they have a younger spouse. A below-average blood pressure also seems to be common among them.'

There is a growing interest on the part of doctors in sex as a contributory factor to good health. It helps those suffering from insomnia, for example, not just because it may be physically exhausting, but because during sex, serotonin, a natural hypnotic chemical which has an influence on our behaviour and moods, is released in the brain, giving us a feeling of well-being.

Pre-menstrual problems are helped by regular sex, and so are headaches, depression and arthritis. Whether for reasons biochemical, hormonal or psychological, good and regular sex can lead to feelings of self-esteem, and this can influence other parts of your life. Dr David Delvin, author of *The Book of Love*, and a leading sex expert, comments: 'A good satisfying sex life with a loving partner is a sound investment for your emotional and physical health.'

Taking physical exercise is another vital key to staying young-looking. Just look at Jane Fonda, Lizzie Webb, dancers such as Natalia Makarova or choreographers such as Gillian Lynne.

Intelligence, too, plays a part in maintaining the appearance of youth says Dr Weeks, who believes there is a connection between intelligence and physical attraction. It could also be a reason why high-powered public figures tend to stay alert and active at an age when their peer group have long given up and retired.

Dr Weeks found that the 'super-young' people in his survey split into two sections – those who feel physically much younger than their age and those who feel mentally much younger. Many fitted into both categories.

'Those who claim to look physically younger than their years tend to have very active lives, to be very socially inter-active,' he says. 'That doesn't mean they work incredibly hard or expose themselves to stress. They just don't give themselves a chance to get bored. They enjoy novelty and challenge in their lives.

Dr Weeks, aged 43, classes himself as one of the super-young. 'It really is in your mind,' he says; 'you have to keep telling yourself, "I'm young and I feel good". It is like a coach with a football team: you must be psyched up every day.'

There is indeed life after 50 and a great many men and women are busily proving it. The 'age wave' is here, in our rapidly ageing population, with more over-40s than teenagers. In the USA, age is a state of mind and that idea is rapidly gaining ground in the UK, too.

Looking young means being supple, not stiff; enthusiastic, not bored. Above all, it means keeping your mind alert and open to new experiences, new ideas. The more you do, the more you are able to do, with mind or muscle.

CHAPTER 1

SAVE YOUR SKIN

Your skin looks soft and plumped out because of its moisture content: it is the key to a good complexion. In fact, skin contains about 70 per cent water, 10 to 13 per cent of which is within the outer corneal layer of the epidermis. The inner, dermis layer of skin, which contains a cell network, collagen fibres and elastin and which keeps the skin plumped out and supple, holds 15 to 18 per cent of the water contained in the entire human body and acts as a general reservoir.

If the moisture level lessens, and the skin becomes dehydrated, it tends to look drawn, dull and lined. You can't hydrate the skin simply by splashing it with water – the skin is 90 per cent impermeable. The hydrolipidic film, a natural emulsion, defends the skin and controls water loss, regulating evaporation and retaining the right amount of water needed.

Although we usually talk about moisturizing for women, men, too, can get dry skin because skin dehydration is not linked with either age or sex, surprisingly. Our basic levels of water in the skin are determined at birth and it is environmental factors – weather, heat and cold – and what we put on our faces that make the difference. It does not vary with age, only with conditions.

Our skin's grease levels vary throughout life but have little effect on the hydration of skin. Problems that are common to skins described as 'dry' also apply to all other skin types, as soon as they are exposed to a dry environment, whether it is caused by hard water and too much bathing, central heating and air conditioning or weather.

Whatever type of skin you possess, skin loses moisture in cold temperatures and when the weather is hot and dry, causing humidity to fall. In such conditions, water evaporates from the surface of the skin more quickly than can be replenished from internal tissues.

Harsh soaps, strong astringents and face masks can dehydrate, removing too much of the skin's natural protective film.

Products we put on the skin also dry it up. It is called 'chemical interference' by dermatologists. Harsh soaps, stringent exfoliators, strong astringents and face masks are the worst offenders and contribute to dehydration because they remove part of the natural hydrolipidic film.

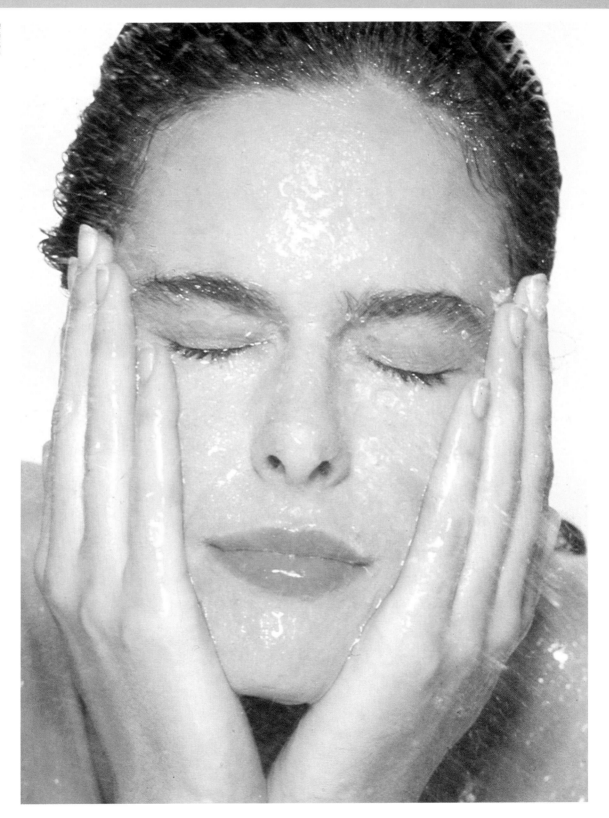

The outer layer of skin, the epidermis, is actively changing every day because of its steady renewal through a process of cellular multiplication. The renewal cycle takes about 28 days. During the first 14 days, cells which multiply in the base of the epidermis re-enforce themselves, spinning a tough protein structure. During the following 14 days, the cells flatten, and eventually rise to the surface and flake off – most of the dust in our homes is actually made up of cast off skin.

At the surface, a good skin looks supple and feels soft to the touch. Its glow, linked to reflection and absorption of light, is luminescent and rosy. But when the skin becomes dry, immature cells may generate a poor quality protein and become damaged, split and porous, and the epidermis will lose its capacity to retain water and protect the skin. The results show in feelings of discomfort, lack of suppleness, roughness and perhaps a scaly appearance, and the skin is dull and pallid in tone.

Moisture is the key

For most skins, and particularly if you want to keep yours looking youthful for as long as possible, moisturizing creams and lotions are an important beauty aid, aiming to copy the skin's own natural protective ingredients. Forming an invisible barrier to stop water loss, they are not just a film of grease, but may copy the skin's own natural moisture-protecting mechanism, and may have other beneficial ingredients such as sun filters.

Normal to dry skins need to use a moisturizer every day. This is usually applied to neck and face, including the eye area and lips. Normal to oily skins may need a lighter type of moisturizer and to avoid using it on the greasiest areas such as nose and perhaps forehead, except in times of low humidity, cold and heat. When the humidity is low, for example when flying, you may need to reapply moisturizer more often.

Some products have longer lasting results than others and the only way to tell which will suit you is to try out different ones for yourself. Emulsions are usually the lightest and creams have more substance, but modern formulations vary from manufacturer to manufacturer.

Apply moisturizer in the morning and allow it to sink into the skin before applying your foundation. At night, normal to dry skins benefit from using a skin cream after cleansing. At one time, these were called 'nourishing creams' or 'skin foods' but this is rather a misnomer because the creams work on the outer, dead skin cells. The living part of the skin is nourished by the blood.

These night creams may have all kinds of fancy names and ingredients but basically, they keep the skin moisturized and supple.

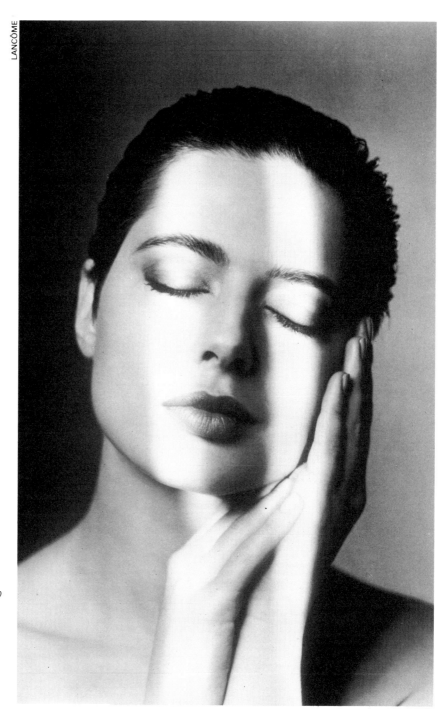

Moisturizing creams help to soften lines and protect your skin, improving its texture. They are a very useful beauty aid but don't expect miracles in terms of rejuvenation.

SKIN PROBLEMS

Few skins could ever be described as perfect. Sometimes it may seem as if your complexion is suffering far too many slings and arrows of outrageous fortune, but there is always something practical you can do to improve matters.

Out damned spot

Somebody once said that if you do something about your spots, they will clear within a fortnight and if you do nothing about your spots, they will clear within two weeks! They were obviously not referring to proper acne, which can be a devastating skin disease that can cause scarring, and should not be neglected.

You would be most advised to see your GP for anything other than the mildest of attacks, because acne today is easily treated and controlled. Acne, the name dermatologists give to spots, zits, or whatever else you call these annoying skin blemishes, is an inflammatory disease of the hair follicles and oil-producing glands and although an excess of grease is linked to it, you can have a greasy skin and still not have acne, so other factors must be involved.

Doctors and dermatologists are still unable to pinpoint the exact cause of spots. However, they are most likely to be caused by an excess of the male hormone androgen, which is present in males, and to a lesser extent, in females. Progesterone, a hormone in the contraceptive Pill, can give androgen effects, too, and may sometimes trigger acne.

How a spot is born Androgens stimulate the sebaceous glands which are attached to pores in the skin (otherwise known as hair follicles) and these produce more oil than necessary. This oil, or sebum, is of a much stickier consistency than that normally produced, and combining with dead skin cells, it may block the pore opening causing a 'blackhead' or 'comedone'. The black colour is caused by the pore opening becoming tinted with skin pigment called melanin (which is also responsible for tanning) which darkens on exposure to light.

In the meantime, oil continues to build up and all this provides the right environment in which bacteria can grow and multiply. When the damned up pore eventually leaks out into surrounding skin tissue, it causes the skin around the blocked pore to become red and inflamed, producing the typical acne pimple.

14

Whiteheads have no opening and so they are not easily unblocked. But, like blackheads, they respond to skin medications and cleansers.

Teenagers may suffer most from skin blemishes, but older skins, too, can have spot problems caused by changing hormone levels, or by products that cause cosmetic acne. Prolonged periods of stress can affect skin condition because of the changed chemical and hormonal influences in the body. Many women suffer from the occasional spot prior to a period or during the menopause and an unlucky 10 per cent of people will still suffer from their teenage acne well into their thirties.

There is a genetic influence, too, and the severity of acne can sometimes be anticipated by how much trouble other family members have suffered. Other factors, such as the use of oily creams, may exacerbate or precipitate acne. If you use a heavy, greasy cream for cleansing, for example (certainly not to be recommended), without using a skin tonic or freshener or soap and water to remove the traces, you could eventually end up with a bad case of acne cosmetica.

The Pill or pregnancy can upset normal hormonal balance, but may also sometimes be beneficial. Diet, however, is thought not to affect acne and dermatologists believe that fatty foods and chocolate are irrelevant. Sunbathing, tradition- ally supposed to help dry up spots, can prove disappoint- ing because after your holiday, you could get eruptions.

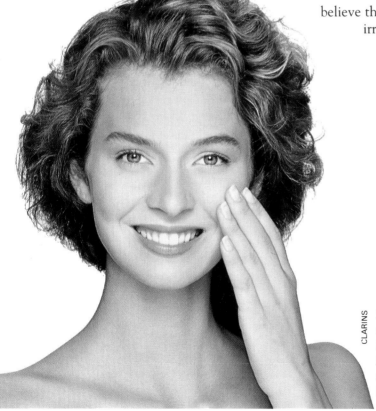

CLARINS

Spots are likely to occur in teenage years triggered off by hormones, but you can get blemishes at any age. Gentle degreasing is better than rougher handling with strong astringents.

This is due to sunlight causing skin to thicken as a protection – this leads to the pores becoming blocked and starting the spot-cycle once again.

Your doctor may prescribe an antibiotic which will need to be taken for months because acne responds slowly, but it is an effective remedy. Dermatologists may recommend a powerful peeling medication based on retinoic acid, a synthetic derivative of vitamin A.

Remedies in the shops   For not-so-bad spots or the odd blemish, over-the-counter spot products are useful. They often contain a chemical compound called benzoyl peroxide. This increases the skin shedding action, and although effective in treating spots, it may sometimes cause overdrying, flakiness, redness and increased sensitization of the skin.

New formulations may contain ingredients such as ethyl lactate and zinc sulphate which affect the acid/alkaline balance of the skin (known as pH) deep inside the pore and dropping it to 4.0 instead of the normal 5.5 level. Bacteria are incapable of living and growing below a pH level of 4.5, thus products containing these ingredients make the pore a very hostile environment, killing bacteria and preventing them from multiplying and growing. This reduces redness and inflammation around the spot quickly and the spots resolve and disappear.

Medicated products help to cut down the bacterial colonization of the skin. Creams, gels and lotions containing ingredients such as benzoyl peroxide or the vitamin A derivative retinoic acid produce peeling of the skin and help to get rid of blackheads. For mild acne, a medicated face-wash can be helpful as an alternative to ordinary soap and water. These cleanse and degrease the skin without overdrying. A medicated cleanser is particularly useful for combination skins – the cleanser is applied to cotton wool and stroked over the greasy areas.

Treatment gels and creams are used for specific spots or spotty areas and should be applied at the first sign of an eruption.

Remember, it isn't dirt that causes acne, so don't be too rough on your skin. All you want is to help reduce surface greasiness. Don't use harsh abrasive exfoliating scouring pads on your face.

Acne rosacea is not like the usual type of acne in that there are no blackheads, but a flush, mainly on cheeks, nose and forehead with perhaps some swelling of the nose. It effects women aged between 30 and 50 mostly, gets worse in the cold and heat and in very humid weather, and after having hot drinks or highly seasoned foods. Emotional stress, too, can trigger it off. A course of low-dose antibiotic is effective.

ELIXIRS OF YOUTH

Famous female film stars are often quoted as saying that they believe love-making is the best beautifier of them all, and even the experts agree that sex is good for beauty. The female hormones are stimulated by sexual activity and this can be beneficial to the skin.

Apart from a regular and happy sex life – and not everyone is lucky enough to be able to count on that – up to now, the ways to make your skin look younger have inevitably involved so-called rejuvenating creams. Whether or not these actually work is debatable.

But when it comes to improving their appearance, people seem to be quite adept at fooling themselves. Plastic surgery patients, it has long been known, are sometimes happier with the results of their face-lifts, eye lifts and nose jobs than their surgeons. And even research into the drug minoxidil, applied to the scalp to encourage hair growth, has revealed that some patients report denser hair growth than seen by their doctors.

The explanation appears to lie in what psychologists call 'cognitive dissonance', the theory that the more time, effort or emotion a person invests in doing something, the more likely she is to believe that the outcome is a success, even if objective evidence points otherwise.

We may feel that any improvement is better than none and in the end it is what we feel that matters. As one doctor commented: 'If a person feels she looks great, who's to argue?'

Rejuvenation – what everyone wants

This is what could well be happening with the expensive rejuvenating creams. They sell hope. The more we spend, the more we seem to believe in the product's efficacy. 'I feel much better when I use an expensive cream,' said one user. 'I feel I deserve the best.' If feeling good helps us to look good so be it. But the truth is that up to now, creams that imply they can turn back the clock (they dare not actually say so because of the advertising code) have probably been little more than expensive moisturizers and lubricants. No sophisticated consumer, let alone scientist, has any expectation that the unattractive results of skin ageing can truly be reversed.

Not that a good moisturizer isn't a good idea: the new generation of

The new 'therapeutic' moisturizers improve the outer layer of skin, the epidermis, and results are much longer-lasting.

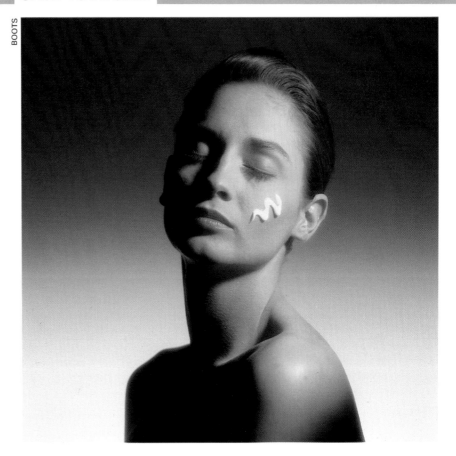

BOOTS

creams go through a great deal of testing in laboratories who can prove that treated skin is softer, has more resilience, looks better in every way. They cannot alter established ageing wrinkles, of course, nor can they put back the clock, though skins look better after using them.

The original moisturizers were occlusive and greasy, and the next type contained humectants, which attract water to the skin surface. When you stopped using them, your skin went back to stage one. The newer, 'therapeutic' moisturizers claim good effects for about 10 days after you stop using them, and that they actually improve the outer layer of skin.

But there is, at last, a medical treatment for skin ageing which could well play an important role in the way we treat our skin, though there are inevitably some side-effects. It has been called the first medically acknowledged anti-ageing cream ever and it is forecast to take us into a whole new area of beauty care.

The University of Michigan has done a double-blind study on the effects of a derivative of vitamin A, retinoic acid or tretinoin, on sun-damaged skin and has presented strong evidence that the wrinkling, sallowness, roughness and mottled pigmentation characteristic of middle-aged and elderly Caucasians who have done a lot of sunbathing, can be improved within a four-month period by daily topical application. Treated skin not only looks younger but seems to act younger, too. New collagen appears to be formed in the dermis.

The side-effect of tretinoin treatment is a slight to moderate dermatitis (redness, tingling and irritation), but this can be controlled with the right treatment. Retinoic acid has long been prescribed by doctors for severe acne, and despite the dryness and scaling of the dermatitis reaction, it has proved to be very successful. Now, it has other uses, but it is still only available on prescription.

Professor Albert Kligman of the University of Pennsylvania was the first to establish the clinical efficacy of tretinoin in the treatment of acne. It was he who first noted the beneficial effect of the compound on photoaged skin (that is, skin prematurely aged by sunlight) and he is so enthusiastic about the treatment that he uses it every day himself. He believes his best advertisement is former US President Ronald Reagan. At his clinic, the Centre for Human Appearance at the University of Pennsylvania, Professor Kligman and his team now see as many men as women.

This whole area raises questions regarding the boundaries between drugs and cosmetics. Tretinoin (trade name Retin-A) is marketed as a drug and appears well on its way to establishing safety and efficacy as a treatment for photoageing.

However, it is hoped that tretinoin is the first but hopefully not the last cosmetic-like ingredient capable of reversing ageing changes in the skin, says Professor Barbara Gilchrest, Chairman of the Department of Dermatology at Boston University School of Medicine, writing in the Journal of the American Medical Association.

Should not the cosmetics and pharmaceutical industries be encouraged to create products truly beneficial to the consumer and separable from lesser products that cannot establish efficacy, she asks? Unless regulatory agencies can define a meaningful intermediate category of therapeutic agents and determine reasonable standards of proof for both their safety and efficacy, the prohibitive cost of new drug development will leave cosmetics manufacturers no choice but the current glib advertising approach to describing their products' value, she says.

Retinoids will probably also have a very important role to play in cancer prevention in the future. Tests have shown encouraging results in treating

19

skin cancer. 'The advent of retinoids is the most exciting breakthrough in treatment of skin conditions this century,' says Professor Gilchrest. They have also proved useful in wound healing and are sometimes used as a pre-treatment five to six weeks prior to cosmetic surgery in the USA.

For us, the consumer, getting hold of tretinoin means seeing a doctor, preferably one who understands the preparation and its side-effects and can give the right strength product and the right kind of advice.

Latest studies have shown that once the maximum benefits of daily treatment have been achieved, the frequency of application can be reduced to maintain improvement, but if you stop using it, you will lose at least part of the gains you have made.

Happily, retinoic acid is not expensive and it should not be a big investment, with a tube used sparingly, lasting about three months, though unscrupulous 'specialists' (special to whom?) may charge an enormous amount for a course.

If you do get a chance to use this treatment for sun-damaged ageing skin, you will need to stop sunbathing and to use a highly protective sunscreen every day because the drug tends to increase the skin's sensitivity to ultraviolet radiation. In any case, as skin ageing is caused by sunlight, it seems rather silly to try to continue if you are using a medication to try to remedy its results.

Professor Kligman believes that you have to lead a shady life if you want to age gracefully. You are most at risk of premature ageing if you are of Celtic inheritance, with blue eyes and fair skin.

Doctors starts patients on .025 per cent retinoic acid cream and if, after using every other day, it doesn't tingle and irritate, a higher dose of .05 per cent may be recommended. Even so, it is to be expected that during the first four weeks, there may be a rosy glow, some dry scaling and irritation, until the skin gets used to the treatment. It takes at least four months of use before you see any positive results. Use cleansers and moisturizers suitable for dry, sensitive skin, and an effective sun filter in sunlight. You may well need to change your usual beauty care preparation to more soothing, non-scented products.

The final conclusions about tretinoin have yet to be written, and British dermatologists, as always, are much more conservative and cautious than their American counterparts. But beauty on prescription with new age 'cosmoceuticals' could well be something we shall be using increasingly in the future.

FACE SAVERS

Skin is the body's biggest organ and if you want to roll back the years, the first thing you have to do is look after it, protect it and cherish it. Soft, clear and elastic when we are young, skin changes at puberty with the encouragement of sex hormones, and that is when we begin to get problems.

If you come from a fair English/Celtic background, you may end up with a fine-pored, delicate skin that hates the sun. A Mediterranean or further East connection will be more likely to give olive tones with coarser pores, but which can lap up the sunshine without so much damage.

Oily skins, which look shiny quickly, and have more problems with blackheads and spots, also seem to age the slowest, while dry, fine, fair skins, which look so beautiful when you are young, can soon line.

Looking after your skin

The answer for both types and the ones in between is to cherish this wasting asset in the best way you can and be consistent about skincare. Neglect your skin and you can look older than your years. Look after it, and you stand more chance of fooling the calendar. How you treat your skin depends on your skin type. Sometimes, this is hard to assess. Obviously, you need to treat your skin according to its needs. If you have a greasy, open-pored nose, and drier cheeks, then you will probably want to use a degreasing skin tonic, but perhaps avoid eyes and go easy on cheek areas. When you moisturize, you can leave out the nose. There's no point in adding more grease to a greasy area.

Just what is a normal skin? One that has fine pores, doesn't have blemishes or blackheads, doesn't have greasy areas or flaky dryness.

Sensitive skin If you have fair, fine-pored skin that reacts to weather, ingredients in cosmetics and skincare products, and has problems in sunlight, then you probably have a sensitive skin and should treat it accordingly.

If you react to a particular ingredient, such as perfume, then you have a skin allergy. This is when the body's immune system seems to turn against something harmless for no particular reason. Sometimes skin sensitivity and a skin allergy go together. But not always.

This skin type is probably best served by the unscented skincare ranges, which sometimes describe themselves as 'hypo-allergenic'. That means less likely to cause allergy, but that is not to say you might not still react to one of their ingredients. Sensitive skins that react quickly to both weather and 'chemical interference' need gentle handling with the gentlest of skin products. Not for you the stringent facial scrubs and astringents.

Oily skins produces an abundance of oil from the sebaceous glands, which are more productive in teen years because of hormone levels. Too much grease on the skin can lead to blackheads and spot problems and so skincare will concentrate on trying to degrease and control.

As you get older, greasiness tends to diminish. The difference between a greasy skin and a combination skin is minimal. Most greasiness is concentrated on nose, forehead and chin, where there are plenty of sebaceous glands. Cheeks tend to be less oily anyway.

Dry skin doesn't have greasy patches and tends to become taut and flaky in bad weather conditions. It may feel parched and tends to line quickly. It could be that your sebaceous glands are not very productive: a thin film of oil on the skin does tend to conserve its water content. Or you may have lower moisture levels which are genetically determined. This kind of skin needs plenty of moisturizing, emollient cleansers and no stringent degreasing of any kind with exfoliators or strong skin tonics.

WASH AND WEAR

Whether or not to lather up tends to bring experts out in a froth but the consensus now seems to be that it is fine to wash your face with soap, or a soap substitute such as a 'non-soap' skin bar, or rinsable cleanser, but use the mildest, non-scented kind of soap and rinse it off the skin very thoroughly. Luxurious, highly-scented soaps are best kept for the body and the bath. Never use a deodorant soap on the face either.

Only the most sensitive and dry skins may not be able to take to soap-and-water washing. Soap is alkaline and this has always been held up to be bad for the skin, which tends to be more on the acid end of the spectrum. But healthy skin can rebound back to a normal acid/alkaline balance within 10 to 15 minutes, say dermatologists.

All skin types tend to feel a bit taut after washing. If it still feels tight and sensitive after about 15 minutes, you should change your cleanser. The rinse-off creamy cleansers are kinder – just apply like a cream but lather up with water and then rinse off. They remove make-up, oil and grime

If you like the feel of water on your skin, and find soap is rather drying, try a rinsable cream cleanser.

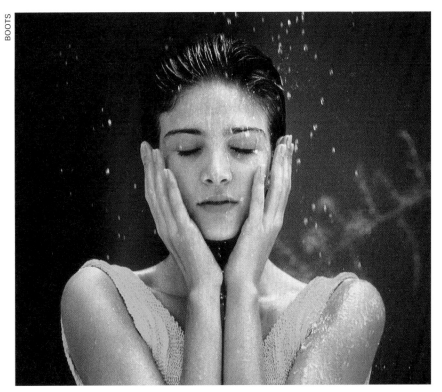

without trouble. If you like to use a face flannel, be sure to put it in the hot wash frequently.

The accepted way to remove make-up (if you don't like soap and water) is to use a make-up remover lotion or cream with cotton wool, followed by a 'rinse' with skin tonic, astringent or skin freshener on another pad of cotton wool.

Take care to wipe off as much of the cleanser as possible with a non-alcoholic, gentle type of freshener, paying attention to round the hairline.

If you find you keep getting spots, it might be a good idea to change your cleanser. Some products contain ingredients that are 'comedogenic' . . . they are more likely to trigger off blackheads (otherwise known as comedones) and blemishes, giving you 'cosmetic acne'. Although long considered the territory of younger skins, this can be an affliction of older skins, too.

Traces of cleanser left on the skin may be irritating. Cleansing creams and lotions, formulated with surfactants, which are a kind of detergent, are not meant to be left on. Add to that some heavy, occlusive, greasy cream, and it would be no surprise to find cosmetic acne is triggered off.

23

Tonics and fresheners are essentially another type of cleanser. The products containing alcohol are stronger, may be labelled astringent, and are more suitable for oily skins. As alcohol is an irritant and very degreasing, it is best avoided by all but the greasiest of complexions.

Alas, no skin tonic or freshener, even the strongest types, can close your pores. Pores are the opening to the hair follicles and they do not have doors that open and close. Tonics are more or less degreasing and may slightly irritate the skin, causing a bit of swelling round the pores and this might have the temporary result of making large pores seem a bit smaller, but they are not 'closing' them.

Eye make-up removal This is best done with a special cleanser on a piece of cotton wool prior to any other cleansing – if you wear contact lenses, choose a non-oily product. This will dissolve the pigments and ingredients without you having to rub. It is always best to treat the fine, thinner skin around the eyes with the utmost respect.

Can cleansing be deep?

The skin is a barrier to the elements and it does a good job of keeping things out. Normally, skin renews itself about every 28 days with new cells 'born' in the basal layer of the epidermis, rising to the surface and flaking off.

If you are too harsh with your cleansing, using too drying products too frequently, you may cause irritation and dryness. But you will be cleansing the outer 'dead' layer of skin – and probably removing too much of the protective skin lipids and natural moisturizers – you cannot go too deeply into the skin with the cosmetic products you buy over the counter.

To describe more abrasive products and skin cleansing techniques as 'deep cleansing' is rather misleading. No cleanser penetrates into the dermis, the inner layer of skin where the collagen and elastic tissue lie, nor would it wish to. Anything that breaches the dead cell-packed outer layer of skin is entering the world of pharmaceuticals, drugs and medicines, and that is a whole new ball game.

So-called 'deep' cleansers are, in fact, 'searching' and include exfoliating facial scrubs, abrasive sponges, face masks and strong astringents. (You can also exfoliate the skin by rubbing with a face flannel.) They are a means of removing some of the outer dead skin cells in order to make your skin look fresher and pinker. Sometimes manufacturers claim exfoliation can speed up your skin cell turnover.

If you rub your skin you cause a small (more or less) irritation. Damage the skin in any way, and it does its best to protect you by trying to grow some more skin cells more quickly than usual. Whether this is a good thing or not is arguable.

As you get older, cell turnover slows down and a build-up of dead skin cells on the skin surface may make an older skin look rather tired and unresilient. A little bit of exfoliating now and again may make your skin look fresher, but don't overdo it. Avoid eye area and lips. If you use a granular type of exfoliating cleanser, rub the granules with little circular movements, and pay particular attention to nose, forehead and chin. Don't think of exfoliation at all, if you have a very fine and sensitive skin.

Dermatologists see more patients who have been far too stringent with cleansing techniques, causing dermatitis, than those who have neglected their skins. Cosmetic manufacturers may talk about stimulation – dermatologists talk about irritation!

Face masks

A mask is a kind of home facial that has a mildly exfoliating action, removing dead skin cells, and leaving the skin looking pinker and fresher. Masks containing clay dry on the skin and are grease-absorbing so they are better for oily skins. Moisturizing masks do not dry into the traditional mask-like effect, are usually transparent, and are best for dry and sensitive skin types. Peel-off gel masks are pretty gentle and mildly cleansing.

It would be misleading to call them 'deep cleansing'. Clay masks are probably more searching than the others. Your face becomes pinker because of the increase in blood circulation to the area, caused by stimulation either by ingredients such as menthol, or because of the clay. When these kind of masks dry, they shrink and pinch the skin so blood rushes to the surface.

Despite all the hype, beauty masks are not a passport to an instant transformation, but can make you feel and look fresher. It's nice to relax in the bath with a face mask occasionally.

For oily skins which have open pores, a weekly clay mask is degreasing and probably beneficial. Other skin types can take a mask occasionally without problems, although you would be wise not to apply one before you go out to a party if you don't want to look too pink. If you have a very sensitive skin and/or broken veins on your cheeks, using any but the mildest of moisturizing masks would be most unwise.

LANCÔME

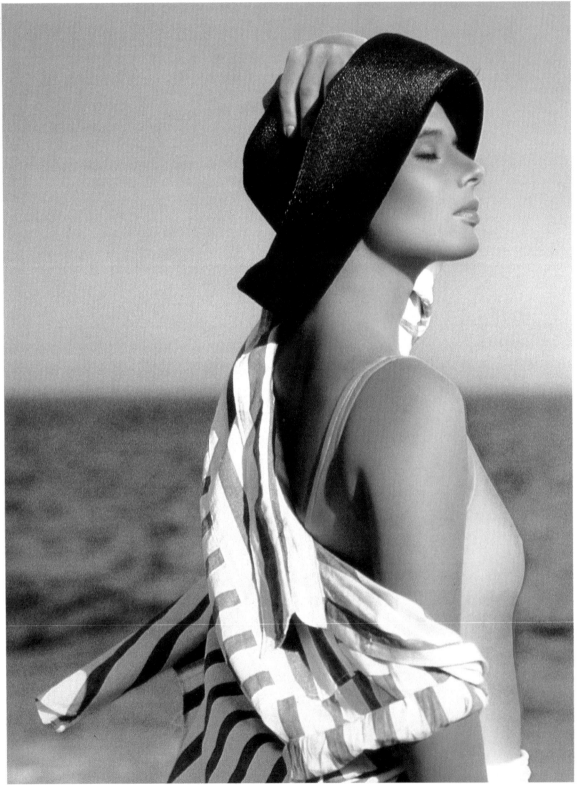

26

DAYLIGHT ROBBERY!

S unlight is a pleasure, but it is also responsible for the big skin steal – robbing your skin of the collagen and elastic tissue which keep it plumped out, supple and young-looking. Above everything else in this book, it is the sun's ultraviolet A and B rays which finally determine whether you look younger or older than the date on your birth certificate.

Long hours spent suntanning on a beach may seem to be doing nothing but give us a glamorous golden colour, at the time. It is later that the cumulative damage done by sunlight makes itself apparent. That's the trouble. At 19, we think nothing (and especially not age) can happen to us. However inside the skin, damage is taking place, and it won't be many years later that the first wrinkles will show up.

The best thing you can do for your skin is not to sunbathe, or at least to use a strongly protective sunfilter that is effective against both UVA and UVB rays. 'But that will slow down my tanning,' you might wail. So it will . . . but it will also slow down ageing.

Jetsetters with unlimited opportunities for sunbathing may expose the skin on their bodies, but are now extremely careful to protect their complexions. The dark brown leathery look is out. A light golden tan is permissible, but the facial glow may well come out of a bottle. However, the message has not filtered through to the rest of us – or we choose to ignore it. New research into suntanning by Windsor Pharmaceuticals, manufacturers of Uvistat, has revealed that around 26 million adults sunbathed last year and of these, 8 million used no sun protection cream whatsoever.

Research proves that people do not understand the sun protection factor system – those numbers you see on sunscreen packs. Although scientists now know more than ever about the long-term health hazards of unprotected sunbathing, and despite the fact that last year the Government ran a £1/4 million national advertising campaign on the need to take care in the sun, the vast majority of people in Britain are still prepared to risk their skin for the sake of acquiring a golden tan.

Fair, Celtic skins and redheads are at worst risk. Those fair-skinned people who live in hot countries can end up with a face that is a fine network of lines all too early, as well as having an increased risk of skin cancer. Olive Mediterranean types, the easy-tanners, have more natural protection but whatever your skin colour or type, your skin will prematurely age given enough exposure.

Sunlight destroys collagen and elastic tissue, and clocks up 'wrinkle time' even in childhood. The sun protection factors (SPFs) indicate how long you can expect to sunbathe without burning (if you tend to burn within 15 minutes, for example, an SPF of 10 would allow you to stay in the sun for 10 times as long). But the factors have, up to now, usually indicated protection against UVB, the burning rays. Look out for products that also protect your skin against UVA, the deep action 'ageing rays'.

If you are not sure of your skin type, you can determine your burning and ageing potential by your eye colour. The palest eyes often go with a skin that makes you top of the risk chart. Extremely dark brown eyes probably go with a skin that is less vulnerable.

A you lose – B you lose

The two parts of ultraviolet light that affect the skin are UVB and UVA. B is for burning: it burns the skin and helps to activate the body's protective melanin, the natural brown pigmentation that gives our skin its tanned appearance.

UVB penetrates the top layers of skin and is not powerful enough to reach down very far into the second layer of skin, the dermis, wherein lies the collagen and elastic tissue. Only about 15 per cent gets through. However medical evidence has proved that UVB damage can cause skin cancers.

A is for ageing. UVA is a powerful ray and although it does not burn the skin as quickly, it helps increase the burning effect of UVB and also penetrates far deeper into the skin, with about 50 per cent reaching down into the dermis. It is thought responsible for wrinkles and ageing. The change in texture to the skin as you get older is due mainly to sun damage from UVA.

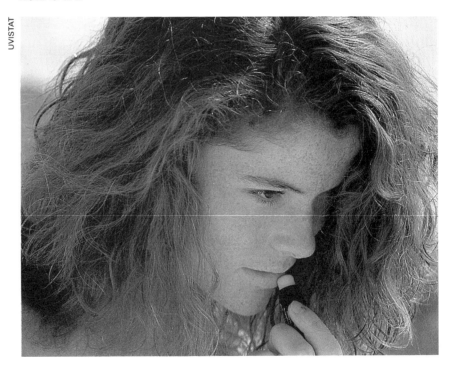

Lips need protecting against sunlight, too. Use a sun protective stick on holiday.

Sun protection up to quite recently has been aimed mainly at UVB. Those sun protection factor numbers you see on packs refer to UVB protection. Some sunscreens do protect against UVA too, but until now, this has been very limited protection. This lack of balance is a bad thing because if a sunscreen filters out a high level of UVB rays but has inadequate UVA screening, it will prevent your skin from burning and allow you to sunbathe for long periods of time, without protecting your skin from the deep-action damage of UVA. You could well be getting far more UVA damage than if you had *not* used a high factor sunscreen, because there is less chance of burning alerting you to the dangers.

It pays to read the label, before you buy. 'State of the art' suntan preparations in the 1990s are going to offer broad spectrum protection against both UVA and UVB rays in a formulation which most closely resembles the balance of the rays in natural sunlight. Higher UVA sunscreens are your best option to stave off ageing wrinkles. The newest anti-UVA chemical ingredient is Parsol 1789. Combined with titanium dioxide it provides an effective screen.

Sunbeds use mostly UVA rays and so accelerate ageing changes in the skin. If you use a sunbed fairly frequently – say three or four times a week – you may develop 'skin fragility syndrome', when the skin blisters if knocked, and bruises easily.

The protection racket

At one time, suntan lotions were advertised as helping you to brown more quickly or brown without burning, but now it is usually the protection they give our skins against ageing which is seen as most important.

Traditional chemical sunscreens, which work by absorbing UV radiation, can, in themselves, cause an allergic reaction in some people. So if you are sensitive, look out for the new opaque reflectant sunscreens which include micronized zinc oxide and titanium dioxide. The particles can now be made so tiny that they are more cosmetically acceptable than before and give a broader spectrum of ultra violet protection, making them the best form of sun protection currently available in the higher factors such as SPF 24.

Micronized protective pigments enable both absorption and reflection, working like an invisible second skin, forming a protective barrier which reflects harmful radiation, but will still absorb enough UV light in order to promote a tan. A good protective sunscreen balances the physical (the reflectant filter) with the chemical.

The solar system

* Do use a protective suncream all the time in sunlight, no matter whether you are an easy tanner or not. Apply it before you go out, and reapply it during the day.

* Remember that on a cloudy or windy day the ultraviolet rays do not disappear, and any cool breeze on the skin may mislead you into thinking you are not getting burned. Even without warmth or in the shade, you can be bombarded with UV light. It is very deceiving.

* How much ultraviolet light reaches your skin depends on latitude and height as well as season and time of day. You will get more UV radiation on the top of Mont Blanc than at sea level. There's most UVB light at noon with the sun overhead, least at dusk. With each 300 metre increase in height, the burning potential of sunlight increases about 4 per cent. So the higher you climb, the more you are at risk of sunburn, and you'll need the strongest protection.

* Sunlight is reflected – about 86 per cent by snow, but also by sea and even by sand to add to the total rays attacking your skin. In water, at least 40 per cent of UV radiation is transmitted to about 20 inches, so you can get burned while swimming.

* If you must sunbathe, avoid the hottest times of the day, between about 11.30 am and 3.00 pm. When the sun's rays are directly overhead, they are most powerful and harmful.

* Sunburn does not peak for about 24 hours. A little bit of red at 4.00 pm can look far worse by 10.00 pm.

* Wind and water cool you down and fool you into thinking it's OK to keep on sunbathing when you should not.

* Never fall asleep in sunlight. You may start in shade but shadows can shift. Have your siesta indoors.

REVLON

30

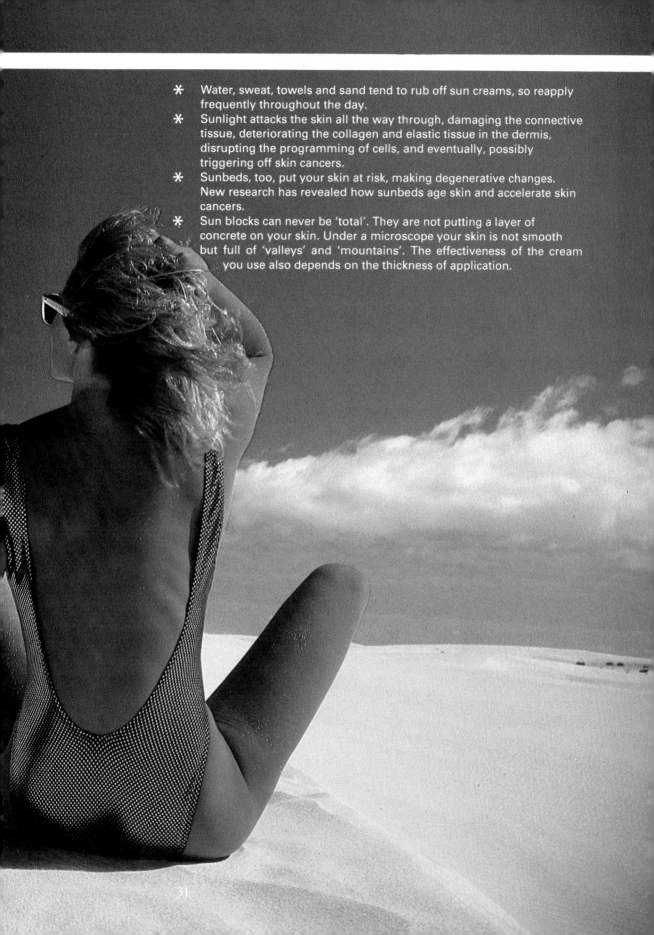

* Water, sweat, towels and sand tend to rub off sun creams, so reapply frequently throughout the day.
* Sunlight attacks the skin all the way through, damaging the connective tissue, deteriorating the collagen and elastic tissue in the dermis, disrupting the programming of cells, and eventually, possibly triggering off skin cancers.
* Sunbeds, too, put your skin at risk, making degenerative changes. New research has revealed how sunbeds age skin and accelerate skin cancers.
* Sun blocks can never be 'total'. They are not putting a layer of concrete on your skin. Under a microscope your skin is not smooth but full of 'valleys' and 'mountains'. The effectiveness of the cream you use also depends on the thickness of application.

UVISTAT

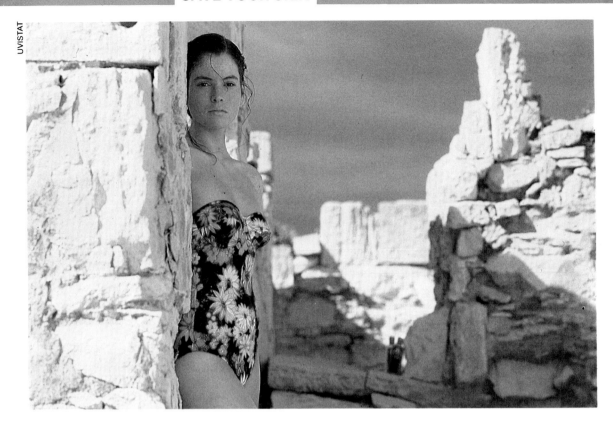

Broad spectrum sunscreens, which protect your skin against both burning UVB rays and ageing UVA rays are the best way to prevent wrinkles. Remember, ultra violet rays reach your skin even when you stand in the shade.

Browning without burning

Can you get a tan if you use a sun filter? The answer is yes, and though you might not get as brown as you want as quickly as you want, it will be better. If you rush a tan you will damage your skin and the tan will peel off quickly. Tanning gradually and gently is best. Use a factor 15 sunscreen, say, which is highly protective, and you can go a light golden brown in two weeks, depending on your skin type (not everybody can get a tan) without visible reddening.

Water resistance is also important. New formulae may contain a polymer which protects the skin from the drying effects of salt water and provide a high level of water resistance for over 85 minutes.

Remember that your tan is adding to your skin protection – a reasonable brown gives you a sun protection factor of about 3 or 4, a deep tan about 5. Add that to the factor number of your sunscreen and your SPF 8 is going to be acting like a factor 12. That's why it seems logical to drop to a lower factor number as you near the end of your holiday if you have developed a tan. But don't forget that you need UVA protection even if you have a tan because the damage and ageing will continue.

A rash result

Up to a third of sunbathers suffer from photodermatosis, an allergic reaction brought on by exposure to the sun. Often incorrectly referred to as prickly heat or heat rash, the condition is primarily triggered by UVA radiation reacting with substances stored in the skin, including antibiotics, artificial sweeteners, fragrances, drugs such as sedatives, citrus fruit and various substances contained in food and drink.

Sun rashes can appear a couple of hours after sun exposure but can last as long as the holiday. If you know you are prone to get them, take extra care. Use a high protection factor sunscreen which is active against UVA as well as UVB rays.

An opaque reflectant is best because it helps to reduce the risk of allergic reactions to sunscreen chemicals. An SPF of 20, a sunblock-type preparation with high UVA protection would be best, though this will also stop you tanning.

Keep out of sun in conditions of intense heat and humidity. Avoid the sun at midday, drink mineral water rather than sweetened soft drinks, and avoid using any product that contains perfume on your skin in sunlight.

CHAPTER 2

LAYING FOUNDATIONS

Cosmetics are the finishing touches few women would want to be without. As aids to confidence, both camouflage and enhancer, they have a long history, but never before have they been so safe and effective, nor has the choice been wider.

The problem is, the choice is so large that it can be bewildering. Just what should you use to make yourself look good and what tricks can make you look younger than the date on your birth certificate?

The older you get, the more you might feel the need to use more make-up but the secret of success is not to let it be noticeable. You can get away with extremes of fashion and bright colours when you are in your teens and twenties. If you are over 40, they can look garish and contrived.

Discreetly applied cosmetics can enhance your looks, whatever your age, and remember the maxim 'less is more'!

If you have been wearing the same shades for years and applying your cosmetics in the same old way, your make-up might look dated, and that can certainly make you look older. So take a close look in the mirror and try to see what is actually there, rather than taking it for granted.

The base of beauty

Unless you have the most perfect skin in the world and beautiful natural colouring, a foundation will be the very pivot of your basic make-up technique. It can cover imperfections, disguise broken veins or dark circles under your eyes, and provides the base for the rest of your make-up.

Blushers are among the most enhancing of cosmetics, lighting up your looks and making you look younger and healthier. But don't be too heavy handed with application.

Choosing the right kind of foundation is usually a matter of testing. In a store, try the foundation tester on your face, not your wrist – take a hand mirror along and inspect the colour in daylight, near a window, not just in artificial light. Try to match the colour of your skin exactly. If you need livening up a bit, that will come later with blusher.

If you go brown in summer, you will obviously have to change your

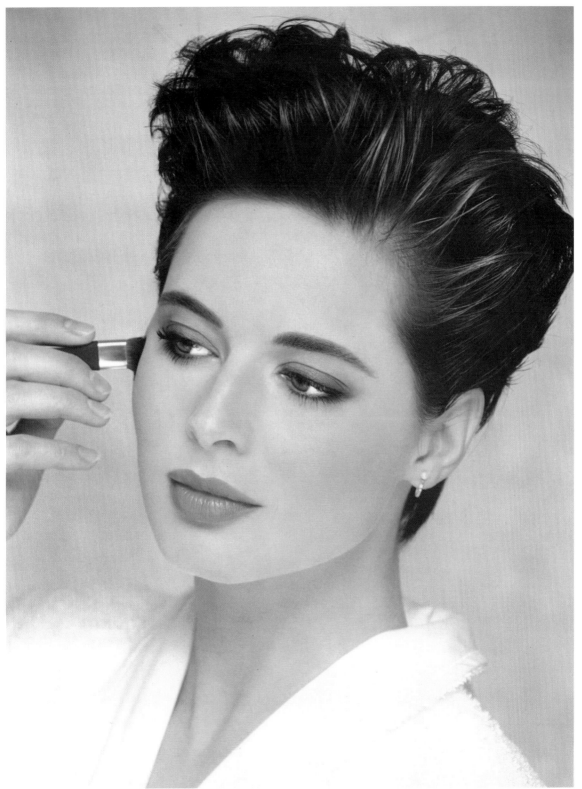

35

foundation shade. Mix a darker shade with your usual one to get just the right colour for your skin. Then you can add or subtract colour to exactly match as your tan fades or deepens.

The kind of foundation you choose will depend on your skin type, how much coverage you want, and how you like the method of application and texture.

Liquid foundation is easy to apply, and give a natural moist finish for normal to dry skins. Apply after moisturizing skin (allow moisturizer time to sink in first) to one section of the face at a time, fading away at the hair and jawline. Follow with a dusting of loose face powder for best results.

New generation liquid foundations are long-lasting, covering but natural. Sometimes silicone-based, they can be lightweight and silky, and many contain a built-in anti-ageing sunscreen.

Oil-free foundations give a matt finish for normal to oily skins. Always shake the bottle well before applying because the contents may settle. Apply sparingly to one section of the face at a time, blending away round hairline and neck.

Mousse make-up is one of the newest methods of application. It gives you an ultra-light, water-based foundation and may contain skin conditioning ingredients. Light and fluffy, it blends in quickly and easily and covers small flaws. You can build up thin layers to get a better coverage if you want. Apply after moisturizing, shaking the canister and pumping a small amount of mousse onto your fingertips, then blend onto one section of the face at a time. Complete with a dusting of loose face powder for a longer lasting finish.

Cake make-up is a matt make-up, comparatively waterproof, ideal for combination and oily skin types; it gives excellent coverage and a matt finish. To apply, saturate a cosmetic sponge with water and then squeeze until it remains damp but not dripping. Rub sponge lightly over cake make-up and apply over entire face with quick, light strokes.

Remember to blend well away under jawline. Next, squeeze sponge out thoroughly and with the clean reverse side, go lightly over the skin again for an even finish.

Cream stick make-up gives the most coverage, and is particularly suitable for normal to dry skins. Quick to use, it cancels out broken veins and skin imperfections. Stroke lightly onto forehead, cheeks, nose and chin and blend smoothly over face with fingertips, blending out to hairline and underneath jawline. Check that it is well blended in around the nostrils.

Cream powder is a creamy blend of foundation and powder in a compact, and it is applied with a puff. Pat gently but firmly all over the face, but don't put too much on. It gives a quick dusting.

Tinted moisturizer is good in summer, when you have a bit of a tan, and is sheer, light, gives a healthy look, but is not usually covering. It will not cover blemishes. Smooth over face evenly and blend into neck. You can set it with a dusting of powder if you wish, or just leave a natural shine.

Powder Tactics

✳ Loose face powder is important to set your make-up if you want it to last as long as possible. Apply it with a clean piece of cotton wool, rolling it gently into skin but not rubbing. Apply powder over foundation and cream blusher if you use it.

✳ Powder eyelids, too, to give a base for your powder eyeshadows. You can use a cotton wool bud dipped in loose powder to set eye make-up or liner and also your eyebrows if you have used a pencil.

✳ Too much powder settling into wrinkles can emphasize them so just 'blot' those areas and brush off surplus. Use a large, soft powder brush to brush away powder, sweeping downwards over the face.

✳ It is best to powder away shine when retouching your make-up during the day with a pressed loose powder rather than a cake powder, which can cause a build-up if you are not careful.

✳ If skin is very greasy (usually on nose and forehead), blot carefully with a tissue first, before powdering.

The beauty of blusher

Pink cheeks and a glowing skin are traditionally the blush of youth, and there's no cosmetic that can give your looks such a lift as blusher.

Powder blusher   Apply with a big soft brush – the smaller brushes that go with a blusher kit are not really big and soft enough and it is worth investing in a good brush because you will find it easier to use.

To apply: smile and find your cheekbones. Look for the 'apple' of your cheek, and dust blusher from the centre of the 'apple' up and out towards the hairline. With your large, fluffy brush, go over this area in circular motions to blend the colour.

Always use half as much colour and twice as much blending – you can always add more colour if you need it. Apply powder blusher over foundation and powder.

Cream blusher   Fingerprint the colour along the cheekbone and blend until there is a natural, subtle glow, with no obvious lines. Apply on top of foundation and under powder.

Mousse blusher   is lightweight in texture, and can be sporty with a subtle, sheer hint of transparent colour, or dramatic, with a more intense application. Designed to glide over moisturizer or foundation.

Gel blushers   (if you can find any) are best on bare skin in summer, for the sheerest hint of colour.

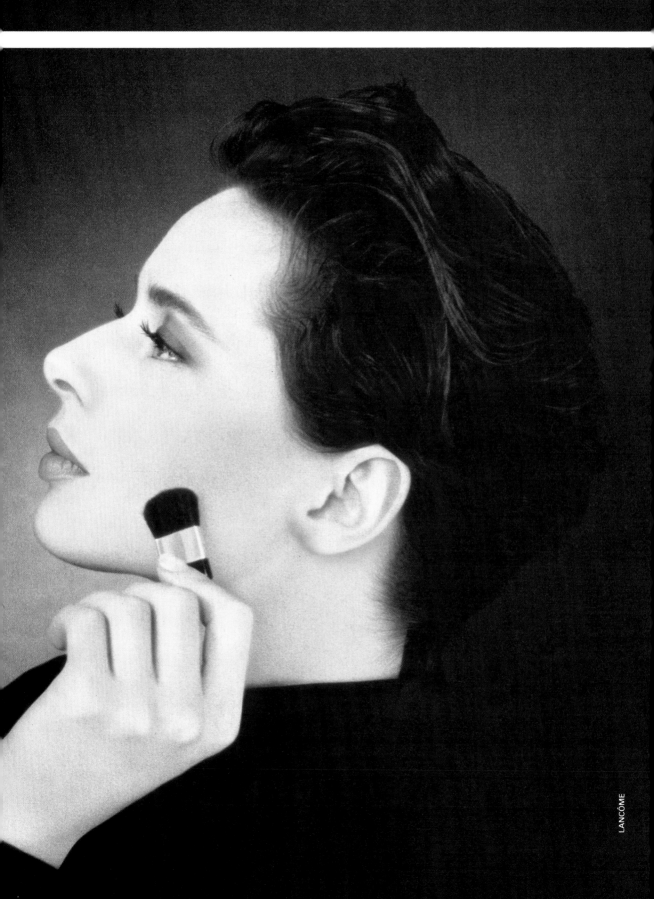

LANCÔME

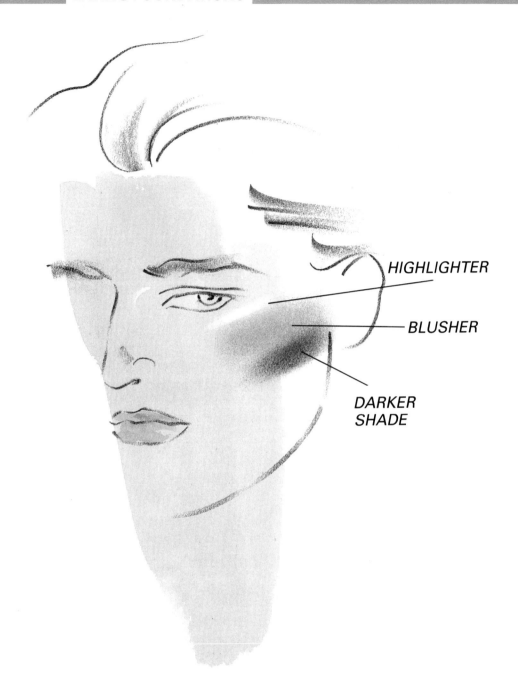

HIGHLIGHTER

BLUSHER

DARKER
SHADE

Evening make-up Make-up can be more adventurous for that special occasion. 'Sculpt' yourself higher cheekbones by fluffing on blusher, then adding a touch of highlighter just below the outer eye, smoothing out towards temples. Contour with a deeper shade of blusher just below cheekbones in the natural hollow (or where it should be).

40

Colours   Whatever the type of blusher you pick, it is best to go for subtle colours: no deep reds, oranges or cyclamens. Strident fashion shades are for those young skins which can afford to take chances.

If you have a pale skin, you'll need a lighter blusher. Dark skins can take deeper shades. In summer, the bronzy powder 'glow' blushers look natural with a tan and are useful for giving you a healthy look all year round – but not with every type of skintone. So you'll need to test it out for yourself.

For a quick make-up, frisk your blusher brush over the eyebone area after you apply it to your cheeks, and whisk it around the hairline at the forehead and temples, too: it is positively therapeutic!

If you look pale and find your blusher simply dies away in the heat in centrally heated houses or in summer temperatures, reinforce the colour by using a cream blusher smoothed on over your foundation, then pat on transparent loose powder, and apply a little more colour with a powder blush in a matching shade, on top.

CHAPTER 3

ALL ABOUT EYES

Eyes are usually the first thing people notice about you and skilful use of cosmetics can certainly make them look prettier. As we get older, the first signs of ageing are usually 'laughter lines', because the delicate and thin skin round the eyes seems to wrinkle quicker than other areas. In fact, some of us have our first wrinkles in our 20s, especially if we have done a lot of sunbathing.

The human eye, says Dr Desmond Morris, is 'the most remarkable organ in the entire evolution of animal life.' The retina has 137 million cells and in fact, your eyes pass 1 1/2 million simultaneous messages to your brain telling you what a person's face looks like.

The iris, which is for adjusting the size of the pupil, appears to have different pigments, but in reality there is only one eye colour in the true sense, says Dr Morris, and that is dark brown. All the other colours are caused by lack of pigment and so blue eyes have very little.

Top: Smoky shades should be subtly applied, blending carefully with a brush, to 'sculpt' eyes and disguise any hooded look. A touch of highlight on the lid can sometimes 'lift' but don't overdo the sparkle.

Dr Morris has pointed out that we like big eyes because babies have bigger eyes in relation to their heads than adults, and having big eyes is a juvenile quality which is appealing. The aim of eye make-up is to enhance the eyes and make them look larger.

We are supposed to have about 200 eyelashes on each eye, though sometimes that seems hard to believe, and they are the only hairs on the entire body that do not turn white when we get older.

Below: Try two-colour shading with lighter colour on lids nearest nose, and smoky or deeper shades on outerlids, shading away up to brow. Deepen next to lashes with liner or darker shadow on a tiny brush for more dramatic emphasis.

The stare, says Dr Morris, is an extraordinary phenomenon: we stare at one another, locking eyes, for two reasons usually. The first is hatred, because staring at somebody is very threatening, and the second is love. We never stare at others when we are not in these moods and the only time you stare at somebody for prolonged periods of time without being threatening is during the process of pair bonding when falling in love.

What is actually happening is that lovers unconsciously check one another's pupil dilation – that shows physical attraction. The pupils get bigger or smaller according to how much light falls on them, like the

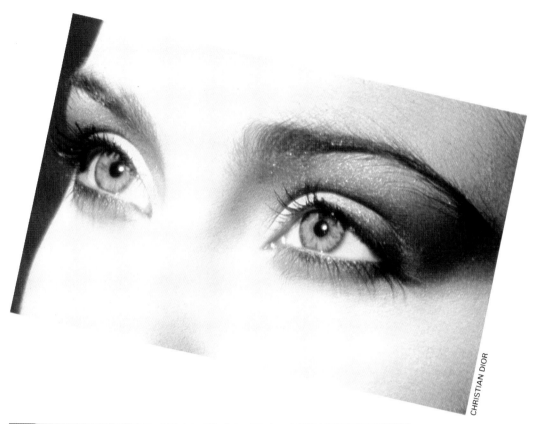

CHRISTIAN DIOR

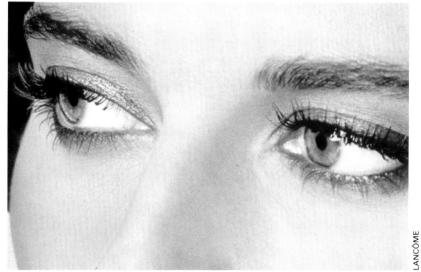

LANCÔME

43

automatic exposure on a camera. But the pupils also become dilated, becoming bigger when looking at someone to whom you are attracted.

Dilated pupils conjure up liking and in advertising, it has been proven that if you artificially dilate the pupils of the model in the photograph, people will buy the product she advertises more freely. Blue eyes are appealing because they reveal pupil dilation much more clearly than dark eyes.

SENSIQ

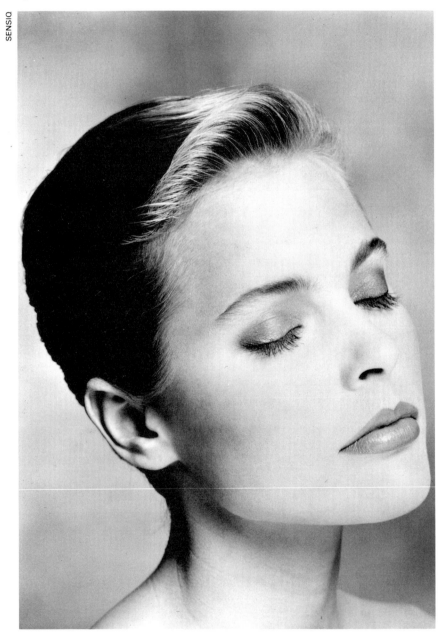

Eye make-up is undoubtedly flattering to most women, but you need to be subtle, not heavy-handed, for a youthful effect.

44

MAKING UP YOUR EYES

Eye make-up needs practice in order to look good – it's not as easy as applying lipstick. If you feel timid about it, try and squeeze a free half hour one evening, and experiment with different types of eye-ideas. Once you get the hang of it, eye-enhancing is quick and easy, and can make a huge difference to your looks.

The trouble is, after many years of doing a particular type of make-up, we may fail to see how we really look. Why not ask your woman friends to give you an honest opinion. I mean honest. You will have to tell them that you won't be insulted if they criticize.

If you want more expert advice, why not invest in a make-up lesson with a qualified make-up artist such as Stephen Glass at Face Facts or those at Joan Price's Face Place (addresses at the back of the book). Going to a beauty salon, where the beauty therapists are not always so expert at make-up application, isn't always a good idea, but if you live out of London ask at your local beauty salon if there is anybody particularly trained in make-up.

If you have pale eyes and fair lashes, eye cosmetics can make you look more definite – bring your eyes right into focus. If you want to lose 10 years, then eye make-up is something you need to master. It is a fashion accessory, a flatterer and a good camouflage.

There is a huge variety of eye cosmetics in a vast array of shades and without experience, you may find it all rather confusing at first.

Eyeshadows

These flattering cosmetics bring colour and shading to your eyes, sculpting a new shape if necessary, enhancing your colouring and your clothes. There are different formulations but these are some of the commonest.

Creams are sometimes oil-based and waxy, come in pots or compacts, and are soft-spreading and easy to blend on the skin with your fingers. There are new formula creams which are less greasy, and longer-lasting. Apply with a finger or brush, on top of your foundation, and powder on top. You can deepen the shade by using matching eyeshadow powder on top of a cream shadow.

Powder eyeshadow is very popular and a good stayer. They sometimes include moisturizers to give cling. In small, flat, pressed-powder

L'ORÉAL

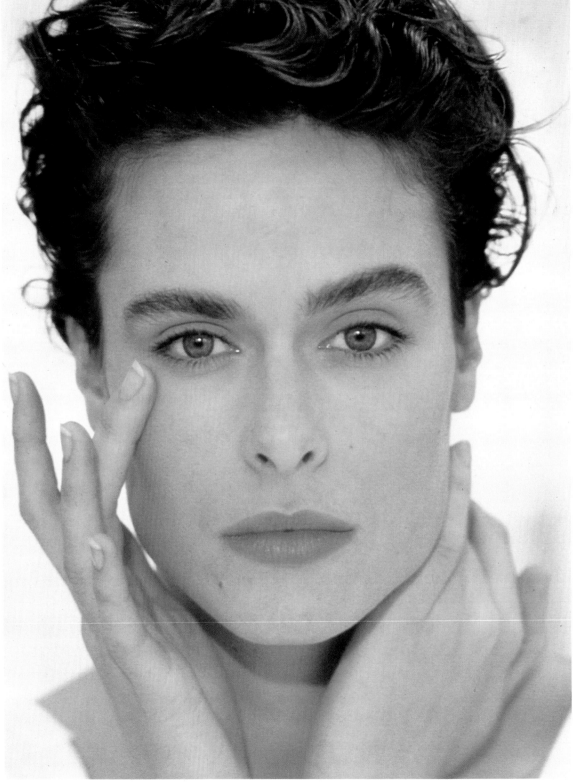

46

Facing page: Make-up looks better on a skin that has been cared for.

cakes or compacts, they come with brushes or sponge applicators, but you will find it easier to control shading with a long-handled sable-headed cosmetic 'paintbrush' or eyeshadow brush. Make-up artists usually prefer to use powder shadows because they give more control. If you want to use a powder shadow as a water-colour, applied with a damp brush, you can indeed do all kinds of blending, but use one side of the block only, if you want to continue with powder application, too.

Sticks are like thin crayons or pencils, and can be harder in texture than creams so they can drag the skin – perhaps not so good when skin is a bit slack and wrinkled. You draw in the colour with light strokes and blend with your finger.

Try off-beat shades of eyeshadow such as subtle browny-pinks, violet-greys, softest khaki and apricot and avoid sparkling bright blues, greens or mauves.

Glosses and gels are creamy and fairly easy to apply and dry to a transparent gleam which is very long-lasting. Not so easy to blend, perhaps, but good for highlighting. They come in little pots, tubes or dipstick applicators. No need to powder on top.

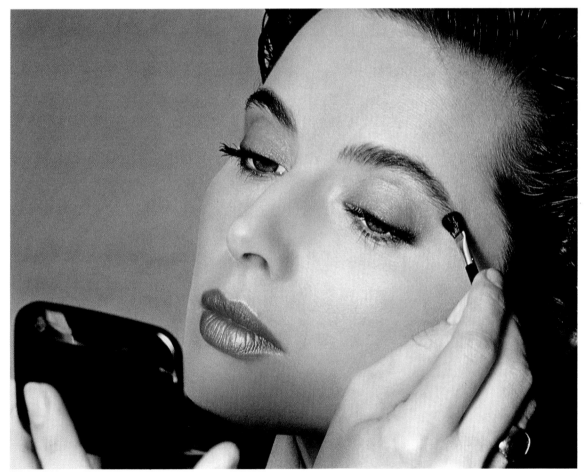

47

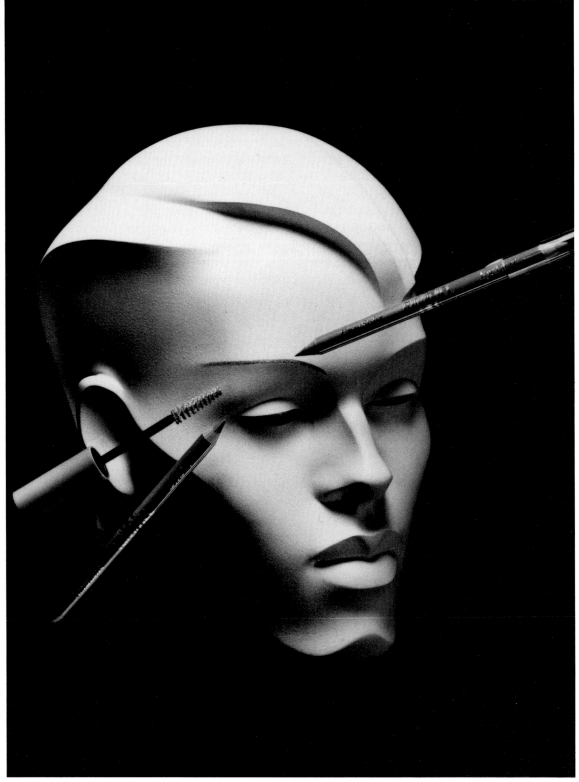

Eyeliners

Enhancing your eyes usually means shading close to the lashes to give the eyes more depth and glamour. You can get the effect using different kinds of cosmetics.

Eye pencils usually have a softer consistency than eyebrow pencils and can be an easy and accurate way to draw the line, but they need sharpening quite often, so invest in the right kind of sharpener.

You may find some pencils too spiky and you certainly don't want to stretch the fine and delicate skin around the eyes. To get more definition, apply a pencil line near to the lashes (half way under bottom lashes, upper lids, or all the way round depending on the effect you want), then use a little brush and matching powder shadow to set the liner pencil and deepen the colour. You can smudge a pencil line slightly to get a more subtle effect if you want, or go round it with a little brush.

Kohl pencils are often very soft and although they were traditionally meant to be used just inside the lower lid in the East, you can use them as a liner, underneath the lashes, too. Applying a dark kohl line just inside the lashes can sometimes have the effect of 'closing' up the eye and making it look smaller. Try it and see for yourself.

Liquid eyeliner comes in a bottle or dipstick applicator and is very long-lasting, but it can make a rather definite line which may look rather hard and stylized if you are not careful. Good for precise, dramatic effects. You need to let the liquid dry before moving on to do anything else with your make-up, or you may get smudging.

Mascara

An important cosmetic because darkening the lashes makes a flattering frame for the eyes. As you get older, it might be better to change from black to dark brown, say, or even grey, to get the subtle effect you want. Try using mascara on top and bottom lashes. If you wear glasses all the time, mascara helps to make the eyes look less 'lost'.

You may not be good at drawing, but it pays to practice your skills if you want your make-up to be enhancing without being too obvious.

Most mascaras are roll-on or brush-on these days. Few of us use the traditional cake mascara which is applied with a dampened brush. Wand mascaras provide automatic application and they are much the easiest to use. Some are thicker than others, and may contain extra fibres or

Mascara darkens and thickens lashes, helping to create a flattering frame to the eyes, bringing them prettily into focus.

filaments to build lash length and thickness. Some are waterproof to withstand swimming, tears and showers. Others are just 'smudge' proof, so as not to leave sooty marks on your cheeks.

Whichever the type of mascara you choose, brush your top lashes downwards and then upwards from underneath to get more of a curl. Brush lower lashes downwards or with a light-handed side-to-side technique. Glued-up lashes that stick together is not the effect you want.

Remove under-eye smudges with a cotton bud – an invaluable make-up aid on any dressing-table. If you use a really waterproof type of mascara, you will need a special eye make-up remover. Avoid any removers with oils if you wear contact lenses.

For a natural look, only wear black mascara if you have very dark hair and darker eyes. Otherwise try brownish-black or just brown. Save exotic pink, green and blue mascaras to just tip the outer lashes for parties – though navy or bottle green can look good with blue and green or hazel eyes, to match your clothes. But bizarre effects are not for you if you want to look younger . . . that is strictly an eye-dea that is best left to the very young.

Eyelash curlers, beloved of many a make-up artist, help to curl up straight lashes and make them more of a frame for the eyes. You place the curlers close to the eyelid with eyelashes inside the two scissor-like halves, eyes slightly open. Close the curler halves together and gently squeeze lashes for about two seconds. Check to see if lashes are curled and repeat if not. But do be careful, because lashes can break off with bad handling.

To make your mascara work for you:

✱ *Do* apply a couple of thin coats of mascara and be careful to separate the lashes. You can do this by careful application or with a dry brush afterwards.

✱ *Don't* use mascara containing filaments if wearing contact lenses.

✱ *Do* go for a hypo-allergenic irritant-screened mascara if you have sensitive eyes.

✱ *Don't* make your lashes so thick and gooey that they look doused in soot. Aim for a more natural look, rather than anything too theatrical, as you get older.

✱ *Do* mascara bottom lashes as well as uppers, for more definition.

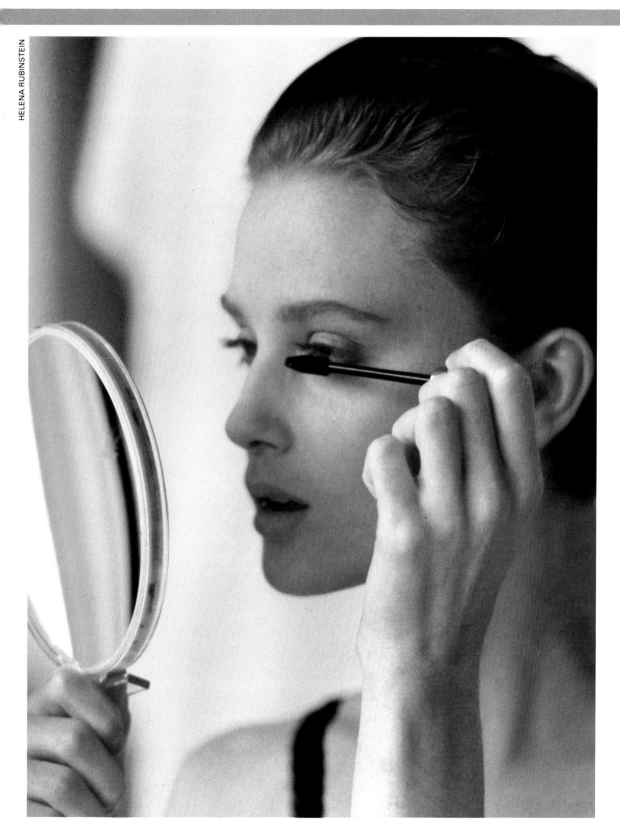

EYEBROWS

I have seen more women look older because of what they have done to their eyebrows than with any other make-up detail. Brows give your face character, and you should never underestimate their impact. Well-defined, *natural*-looking brows are what you should aim for. Nothing makes you look older than peculiar brows – drawn in a fine, thin line, say, in an unbelievable shape, or winging away at the outer corners like a mandarin in a school production of Gilbert and Sullivan. Like the Greeks, the Romans thought that eyebrows which met over the bridge of the nose were a mark of beauty. That is not the case today.

Whatever the fashion, you don't want to end up looking like a plucked chicken. The trouble with plucking is that years later, when you want to have thicker, more natural-looking brows, the hairs don't grow back. The hair follicles just give up the unequal struggle.

If your eyebrows are thick and straggly,   do not make the mistake of over-plucking. Use chisel-edged tweezers, the best you can afford. Automatic tweezers are best left in the hands of beauty experts – they do not seem all that easy to control. Pointed-ended tweezers can prick your skin.

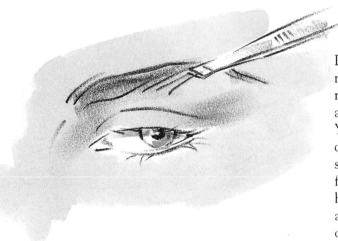

Plucking can be painful for some but not others. If you are sensitive, try rubbing an ice cube over the eyebrow area as a sort of local anaesthetic. You may find it easier to pluck the odd eyebrow after your bath. Or to stretch the skin slightly between two fingers. Pluck in the direction of the hair growth, one hair at a time. Rub an ice cube over the area afterwards, or dab on antiseptic.

Tweeze out odd hairs which grow between the brows and tweak out the odd straggly hairs from underneath the brows, but never from on top. Never overdo the tweezing because you can end up with a permanently surprised look!

Too thin brows because of Nature or over-plucking? You can fill out spaces or add definition with a well-sharpened eyebrow pencil. Do not draw one thick, hard line, but try to do tiny strokes. Don't choose black unless you have black hair, very dark eyes and dark brows and lashes. Otherwise try shades of brown. Blondes with fair skin may find a soft grey and light brown pencil mixed together gives the most natural effect.

Brush-on eyebrow colour is like a block of eyeshadow powder with a short, stiffish-headed brush. Or you can use eyeshadow with a brush, too. You can set eyebrow pencil or tone down any eyebrow cosmetic with a touch of face powder. But pat, don't rub.

How long should your eyebrows be? Try this old make-up trick: Hold a pencil against the side of your nose, the pencil point will indicate just where your brow should begin. The other end of your brow is found by swinging the pencil in an arc until it touches the outer edge of your eyes. Where the pencil point crosses the brow will indicate where you should pluck odd hairs or use pencil.

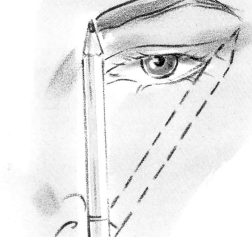

MAKING THE MOST OF YOUR EYES

Eye cosmetics not only colour your eyes, but can re-shape them, too, sculpting with shadows and highlights, making small eyes look bigger, and prominent eyes less bulging.

There is not just one eye colour that is right for you. In fact, using a number of eyeshadow shades, well-blended, can be far more subtle and interesting. Whatever your hair colour, you can wear just about any shade of eyeshadow you choose, depending on where, how much and how you apply it.

The effect you are aiming for is an enhancement of *your* looks, not a clever make-up. In the end, sometimes the last thing you want anyone to notice is that you are wearing make-up at all.

With eyeshadows, the basic rule is: pale colours highlight and 'bring out' making the area seem more prominent and noticeable, and darker colours make an area recede and much less obvious. In much the same way, irridescent, pearly or shiny shadows enlarge and draw attention while matt shadows play down.

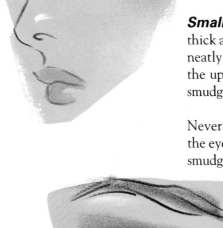

Prominent eyes are less bulgy   if you use deeper shadows on the lids and in the eye socket and highlight the browbone. Stick to matt shadows on eyelids. Use an eyeliner close to lashes to minimize a heavy top lid.

Small eyes look bigger   if you pluck some hairs from underneath very thick and shaggy brows to give more space. Make sure eyebrows are shaped neatly but do not make unnatural arches. Wear a pearl or pale shadow on the upper lid with a touch of highlight under the brow. Brush a slightly smudgy deeper shade just above the eye crease and blend well.

Never use a thick all-round-the-eye liner because it will tend to 'close up' the eye and make it look smaller. If you use a liner, keep it fine. Do a fairly smudgy, subtle shading underneath the lower lid, from half way to the outer edges, and blend upwards and outwards. Mascara top and bottom lids.

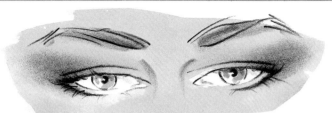

Eyes look further apart if you blend your eyeshadow upwards and outwards. Apply liner pencil or a powder shadow in a deeper shade half way along the top and bottom lids and blend outwards, extending at the outer corners and blending into eyeshadow. Fade away line towards inner corners of eyes. Mascara is most important, especially those lashes at the outer edge of the lids.

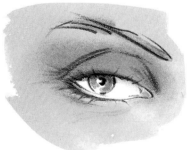

Droopy eyes get an uplift if you brush shadow upwards and outwards at the outer corners of the eyes. Stop any liner before outer edge of eyes and make sure eyebrows do not droop at outer corners. Add a touch of lighter shadow on inner lids, nearest to nose. Blend well. Mascara lashes, especially at outer edges.

Deep set eyes are less sunken if you lighten the eye area, especially if you have dark shadows, using a camouflage cream under eyes. Blend into foundation. Use paler shadow on the lid, taking it higher than the natural crease. Apply a touch of highlighter to centre top lids. If you have a bulgy browbone, shade it down with a subtle grey shadow.

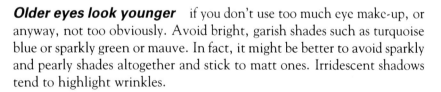

Older eyes look younger if you don't use too much eye make-up, or anyway, not too obviously. Avoid bright, garish shades such as turquoise blue or sparkly green or mauve. In fact, it might be better to avoid sparkly and pearly shades altogether and stick to matt ones. Irridescent shadows tend to highlight wrinkles.

Brown shades may be too much of a good thing – try the effect of a pale and subtle grey, or even a touch of subtle pink or peach, and use wine, navy or grey for definition rather than black.

Be sure to use a soft brush to remove surplus face powder especially round the eye area so powder doesn't end up settling in creases.

GETTING INTO FOCUS

Vanity is the most common reason spectacle wearers give for switching to contact lenses – although they are better for sports such as jogging, tennis, skiing and horse riding.

About half the British population is long- or short-sighted but what is less known is that between the ages of 45 and 65 nearly all of us develop a condition known as presbyopia: we can see distant things but have difficulty in focussing on those nearby.

Like wrinkles, it is, alas, a sign of ageing – the word is derived from the Greek 'presbys' (old man). It is caused by loss of elasticity in the eye lens. When we are young, the eye muscles push and pull the eye, changing the flat shape of the lens needed for seeing distance, to the rounder shape needed for near images.

The near or far images are then thrown on to the retina. But in middle age the eye lens becomes stiffer and the ciliary eye muscles do not work so effectively. The older eye cannot make the instant switch from distant object to near object.

Contact lenses   The solution, up to now, has been to have different pairs of glasses, half glasses or bifocals, with a two-part lens. But if you don't like wearing spectacles, you can now get contact lenses that solve the problem. There are various types of bifocal lenses and one of the newest involves a technique called image enhancement therapy.

A different kind of lens (aspheric in shape, rather like a soldier's tin hat, round at the top but flattening out towards the edges) is specially shaped to intercept rays of light from the nearby object and realign them so the light rays meet the eye's lens at a more gentle angle. This has the effect of helping the eyes to cope, without defocusing, with any object between infinity and about 40 cm in front of the face.

The more usual kind of contact lenses now come in a variety of guises: hard corneal lenses are the cheapest to buy but the most difficult to get used to; gas permeable lenses let oxygen through to the eye so reducing irritation; but soft lenses, though more expensive to look after, are often considered the most comfortable to wear and the easiest to become accustomed to.

Low-water-content soft lenses are the cheaper version and are easier to wear than hard lenses. High-water-content lenses (capable of containing up to 85 per cent water) are very easy to wear but need a lot of care and are the most expensive to look after. The disposable soft lens is worn for a week and thrown away.

Long-wear lenses are increasingly disapproved of by consultants because of starving the cornea of oxygen. It seems sensible to wear lenses for fairly limited periods, look after them impeccably and switch to glasses now and again to give your eyes a rest.

Doctors, who often seem to approve of the hard or gas-permeable lens rather than the soft lens, say regular check-ups with a competent practitioner are essential, at least once a year.

If You Wear Glasses Eye make-up is important for added definition behind your lenses. Apply as much make-up as you would if you were not wearing specs, but it would probably be better to use matte shades rather than anything too sparkly.

Slightly shaded lenses are flattering because they disguise wrinkles, bags and anything else you want to hide, and are also useful if you are short of time to do your usual make-up.

Use a highly magnified mirror for applying eye make-up if you are short-sighted, or you can buy special 'make-up specs' which are designed with lift-up lenses.

Eye savers

✳   Don't smoke – it is a sure way to get premature wrinkling.

✳   Check with your optician to see whether you need a change of prescription.

✳   Try lying down with your feet up and pads of cotton wool soaked in cold, refreshing witch hazel over your eyes.

✳   Or use slices of cucumber or even used, cold, damp teabags!

✳   Relax for 10 minutes.

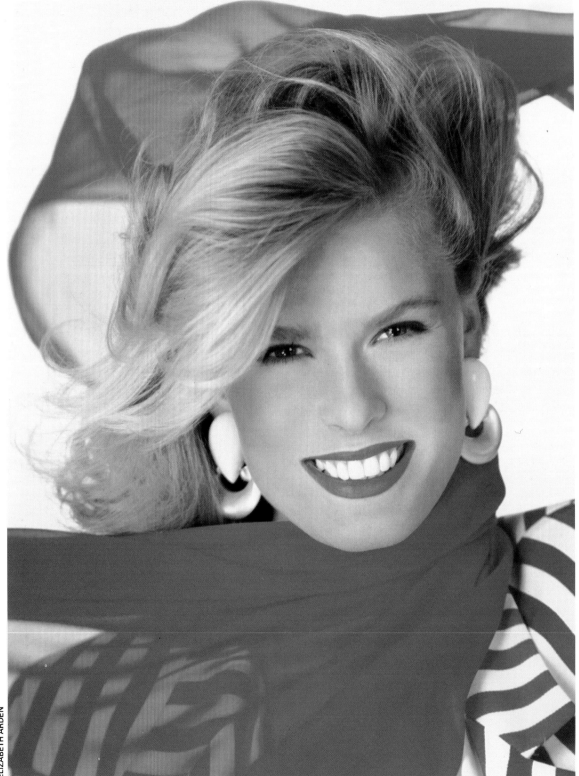

CHAPTER 4

LIP SERVICE

The lips of youth are rosy tinted, and so lipstick has always been a key cosmetic for every woman who wants to look brighter, more alert and youthful.

Lipstick – or rather lip rouge – was found at Ur dating back 5000 years. It must be one of the oldest of cosmetics and also the most popular. It is still probably the last thing a woman puts on before she leaves the house, and although it is just a fairly simple stick of coloured grease, the way you apply it can improve your looks.

Putting on your lipstick seems to complete the change from your private, casual life at home to the exposure and formality of public life outside. Its effect on a woman's morale was not underestimated even during the Second World War when some priority was given to seeing that enough lipstick was produced to meet the demand.

Lipstick not only enhances your looks: it is almost like a fashion accessory because the colour you choose will be in keeping with the colour scheme of your clothes. It also acts as a protection to stop your lips drying out in bad weather conditions.

If you find your lips swell up when you use a particular lipstick, it might be because you have an allergy to one of the ingredients, and most usually, the perfume. You might be allergic to the colouring pigments or a preservative such as paraben, which is also known to be a sensitizer. Leading hypoallergenic cosmetic ranges usually eliminate all known sensitizers from their products.

A crisply drawn mouth, without blurred edges, looks younger and smarter. Try under-lipstick anti-'bleed' treatments, draw the shape with lip pencil before filling in with lipstick. Don't overdo the gloss.

Youth-proofing your mouth

Peeling and dry lips can happen at any age. Health, diet, steam heat, sun or just central heating or night-dryness caused by evaporation of moisture, can cause flaking and lips get dry and chapped quickly in cold weather. Prevent loss of moisture by using a lip balm or salve fairly frequently – under your lipstick or worn by itself. Moisturize the lips at bedtime to keep them supple and smooth while you sleep.

Moisturizing lipstick control or fix products combine a treatment base, fixing agent and priming product in one. The cream softens and moisturizes the lip surface and by helping to minimize fine lines around the mouth, it helps the problem of lipstick 'bleeding' – a boon for the more mature woman or for anyone wearing strong lip colours.

Lipstick has a waxy base and new ingredients which might be added to the waxes and tints might be polymer, which adheres to the skin and fixes the colour, silicone, vitamin E and allantoin to help soften and heal the skin. This kind of formulation helps prevent 'feathering', 'bleeding' or 'running', when lipstick spreads outside the lipline up the tiny lines around the outer edge of the lips . . . a very ageing kind of make-up problem.

If you find your lipshade tends to change colour on your lips, it might be due to the acidity in your skin. Use foundation and powder to prepare your mouth before application.

What colour to choose depends on your likes and dislikes and the colour of your clothes but try to experiment rather than reaching for the same old shade, year after year. As you get older, softer and more subtle lipstick colours are kinder to your looks. Strong deep reds or magentas may draw attention to lines around the mouth, and if your lipstick 'bleeds' into the fine lines, it will be more noticeable with a strong colour.

A lipbrush helps you to define the lips crisply and accurately, and you can use up stubs of lipstick economically. Make-up artists swear by them, but most of us just use the lipstick by itself.

To help your technique, seat yourself by a mirror, balance your elbows on a hard surface and rest your little finger against your chin to stop any wobbling. Hold your wrist with your other hand as you hold the brush between thumb and forefinger, low down near the bristles, for stability.

A lip pencil shapes, shades, outlines, fills in and makes lipstick really last. For anti-feathering, the pencil formula lays down a matt colour barrier to prevent lipstick from creeping. If you have a lot of lines, apply your lip pencil, then powder over the pencilled area lightly. Now apply lipstick, stopping the colour just short of the mouth edges.

Lip gloss can add gleam for day, shimmer for evening. Apply with fingertips or brush over lipstick, or use alone for intense shine and subtle colour. You can put gloss all over, but it is preferable to apply it to the centre of the lips to intensify the lush, shiny look of any lip colour and provide protection against dryness and chapping. Too much gloss, however, will soon wear off . . . taking the lipstick with it. Don't be too heavy handed or your mouth will look jammy.

Best way to shape up your mouth

* If you have a problem with 'bleeding' use a special lip-fix product on the lips first. This helps the lipstick to stay put.
* Outline your lips with a lip pencil which must be sharpened to a fine point and the shade chosen to blend with your lipstick colour.
* Put two pencil dots on the upper lip at the highest points of your cupid's bow. These dots will guide in shaping the upper lip. Now, with the mouth closed, start by drawing a 'V' shape with a line from each dot downward to the centre of the mouth. Outline from each dot to the outside corners.
* On the lower lip, outline from the centre to the outer corners.
* Apply lipstick to the upper lip first, then the lower lip. Fill in the outline, preferably using a lipbrush for best results.
* If you use the lipstick directly from the tube, never swivel it all the way up and never use a lot of pressure. Just glide the colour on.
* Two light applications will look prettier and smoother than one thick one and will lessen the chance of colour change. Some make-up artists say blot the lips inbetween coats for longer-lasting results, and apply foundation and powder over the lips first, before you begin. But other make-up artists advise not blotting your lip colour because it takes away the colour quality and shine. Try each method out for yourself to see which suits you.
* Always remove old lipstick before reapplying.

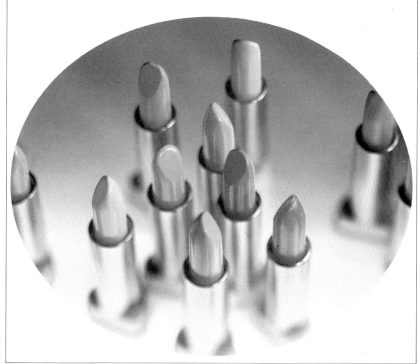

BOOTS

61

Lip corrections

You need to practise these kind of make-up tricks carefully to get them subtle. For any mouth that needs correction, first cover with foundation and powder to blot out the original shape.

Too full lips get slimmed down by using lip pencil to draw the mouth shape just inside the natural lipline, defining the outside corners well. Avoid colours that are too light, or too bright, shiny or frosted, because they will accentuate the fullness. Apply a medium lipstick shade extending to the outer corners of the mouth.

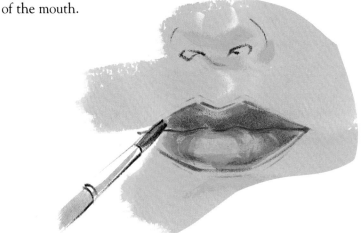

Too thin lips look a little fuller if you use a lip pencil to outline slightly just beyond the outer edge of the natural lip line. But go easy here because if you are too ambitious the result will look unnatural. Dark shades will make lips look thinner, so use light to medium colours and shiny or frosted shades and lip gloss.

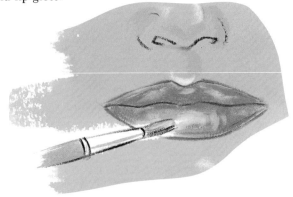

Too wide mouth: use lip pencil to outline but stop just inside the corners of the mouth. Fill in with a slightly darker shade of lipstick.

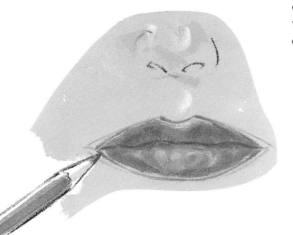

One lip fuller than the other: emphasize the top lip by using a lip pencil slightly beyond the outer edge if it is thinner than the lower lip. Then apply a light, bright colour of frosted, shiny lipstick, topped with gloss. De-emphasize the fuller bottom lip with a toning but deeper colour and don't use gloss on it. A dot of pearly highlighter in the dip of a cupid's bow or the centre of a bottom lip will help to create the illusion of more fullness. Try using gloss on the thinner lip, blot matt the fuller lip.

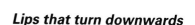

Lips that turn downwards at the corners? Do not take your lipstick colour into the lip corners and try to draw a more cheerful shape by lifting very slightly and subtly at the sides. Try using a lip pencil first to get it right.

A BETTER BITE

Your teeth can make an enormous difference to your looks, especially as you get older, and it is worth all the effort and expense to get them right. If you cannot smile because of crooked teeth, have unsightly gaps, or discoloration, then you are short-changing yourself and your appearance.

Take care of your teeth and you can hang on to them for as long as possible. But if there are problems, you need a dentist who is interested in conservation and aesthetics . . . and not all dentists are skilled in reconstruction dentistry with capping and bridgework.

Now there are other possibilities, too, with veneers and new bonding agents. If you lose teeth, your face can become more sunken and that can certainly make you look older.

Having your teeth fixed can do a great deal for your confidence, but it is your own personal dental hygiene which will help to keep them longer.

Plaque is the sticky substance responsible for both decay and gum disease. It is made up of millions of bacteria that grow on gums and teeth and accumulate between the teeth and at the gum margins. This plaque is always there, more or less, and needs careful and patient removal every day in order to stop future problems.

The bacteria in the plaque makes acid as it feeds on sugars in the mouth and the acids attack the tooth enamel, while toxins made by the bacteria cause gum edges to become inflamed and enlarged, leading to pockets where plaque can collect. When plaque is not well enough removed, it hardens into tartar which is not removable with normal toothbrushing. As pockets get deeper, there is the danger of getting abcesses, and eventually teeth loosen and fall out or will have to be removed. This can change the shape of your face and contribute to a sunken look. The best way to stop trouble is to cut down on sugar.

Use disclosing tablets to stain plaque so you can see just what you are brushing. Try using little 'flu-brush' interspatial brushes with tufts that can clean between the teeth, and try changing your normal toothbrush regularly. You'll need at least four a year.

The best brushes are multi-tufted with rounded filaments to prevent gum damage. Mouthwashes are just a temporary measure and only mask bad breath for a little while, without tackling the cause. Better invest in regular hygienist treatment at the dentist to steer you onto the right track.

CHAPTER 5

TAKING STEPS

If you want to roll back the years, albeit temporarily, there's no doubt cleverly applied cosmetics can give a great boost to your looks. It pays to learn to be your own expert make-up artist, becoming adept at camouflage, subtle with colouring and skilful of technique.

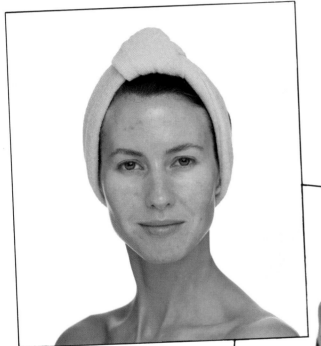

Bare faced . . . spots, blemishes and uneven colouring.

Beautifully made up . . . gently enhanced, blemishes camouflaged.

65

PRIMING THE CANVAS

1 Apply a light moisturizer and allow it to sink into the skin for at least 10-15 minutes before you apply any make-up. Avoid anything too oily.
2 A concealer stick or cream disguises spots, under-eye shadows, uneven patches of redness. You can apply a little more later, if necessary, over foundation and blend away edges.

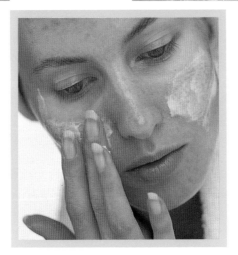 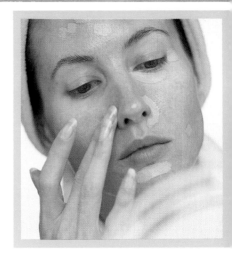

BRUSH STROKES

5 A big, soft powder brush is useful for brushing off surplus powder.
6 It's better to use a big, soft brush, too, for applying blusher, which is one of the most flattering cosmetics for lifting your looks. Apply from centre cheek and sweep upwards and out to temples. Don't be too heavy-handed.

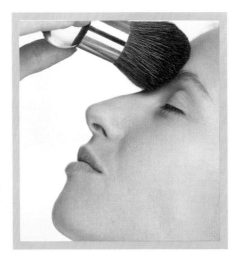 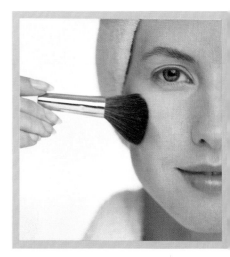

FINE DETAILS

9 Apply charcoal grey shadow to outer corners of eyes and blend up into socket.
10 Dust a paler, touch-of-gold shadow on the lids – but nothing sparkly. An earthy brown colour defines the eye socket, and will help to disguise any hooded effect. If crepey lids make eye colouring more difficult, lift lid gently with finger.

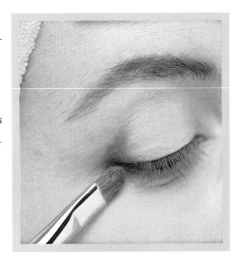 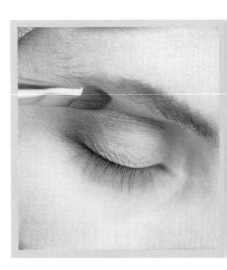

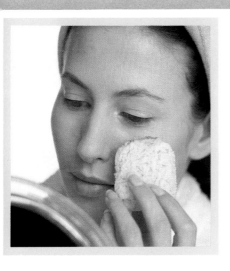 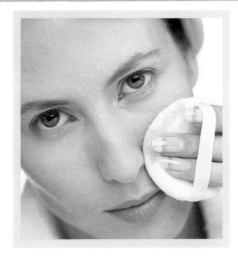

3 Apply skin-matching foundation with fingers or a small sponge. Blend away carefully round hairline and under chin.
4 Loose powder sets your make-up and keeps it looking fresh for longer. Pat it all over your face with a puff or a ball of cotton wool. Use a lighter touch around eyes where powder can settle into wrinkles.

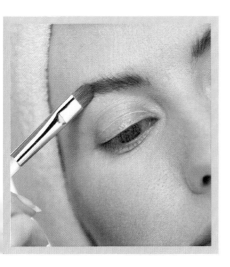 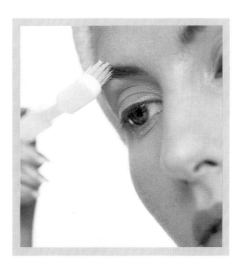

7 Define eyebrows with pencil or use eyeshadow powder on a brush for softer touch. Avoid over-plucked arches or exaggerated sweeps which always look ageing.
8 You can soften brow colour and remove surplus powder with a brush – a baby's toothbrush will do. Colourless mascara is useful for brow grooming when hairs get straggly.

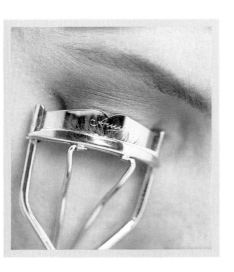 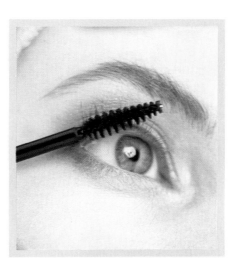

11 Eyelash curlers are useful if you have naturally straight lashes. Use them before applying mascara.
12 Apply a couple of thin coats of mascara and go over lashes with a clean brush to stop clogging.

FINISHING TOUCHES

13 Use a lip brush to outline mouth for a younger, crisper finish.

14 Finally, fill in with lipstick.

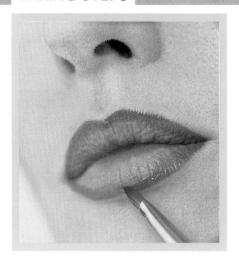
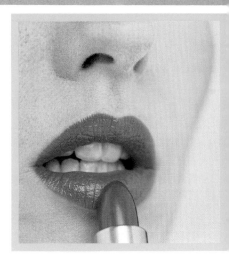

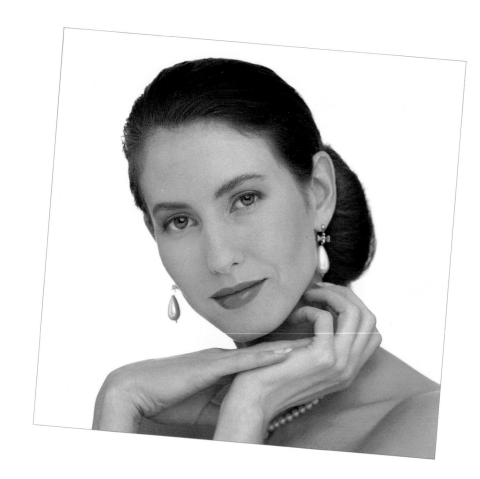

CHAPTER 6

ARTS & CRAFTINESS

The one rule of today is that there are no real embedded-in-concrete rules anymore, only what is right for you and your particular looks. That goes for beauty, hairstyles and clothes.

Nobody's perfect, nor is that the aim of your make-up techniques, but there are skilful ways you can enhance your best points and minimize anything you think detracts from them.

We have borrowed from stage make-up with its magic tricks of light and shade, but you have to use a lighter hand and remember that what can look good in artificial light may look dreadful in stark daylight.

Here's how you can borrow some of a make-up artist's skills . . .

Give your skin luminosity by using a porcelain pale underbase to cover flaws, and top with your usual foundation.

Soften wrinkles by using a moisturizer before you apply your base. Make skin matt with face powder, but not too much and be careful not to let any set in deep wrinkles. Avoid any metallic or pearlized cosmetics as the sparkle can settle into wrinkles, draws attention to them, and can make them look deeper.

Beat the blushes by using a colour corrector cosmetic, or underbase worn underneath your usual base. This is usually a very subtle pale *green*, and it does seem to work.

If you have red-veined cheeks, avoid red or mauve blushers. Keep blusher away from the over-rosy part. But if you apply a camouflage, you can still wear blusher, and this way you get the colour where *you* want it.

A camouflage or concealer stick or cream can be used over or under your foundation over the bits of your face that usually go red (nose, cheeks). Your foundation should be non-pinky, of course, preferably in a beigey shade, then dust transparent loose powder on top to set.

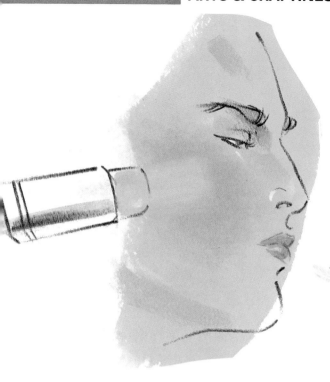

If you go pink with even a single drink, or flush up in the heat of the kitchen because you have naturally high colour, try a touch of concealer cosmetic to tone you down. Cream stick make-up is particularly covering.

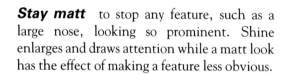

Stay matt to stop any feature, such as a large nose, looking so prominent. Shine enlarges and draws attention while a matt look has the effect of making a feature less obvious.

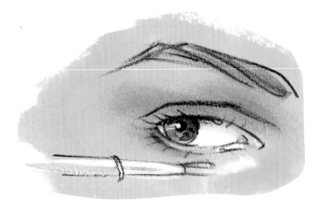

Blot out bags with concealer. Appl[y] cream concealer (or lighter shade of foun[da]tion) underneath the eyes. Apply to the [dar]kest area, just below the tear duct, near [the] nose, and blend away, outwards. Keep pow[der] to a minimum here, to avoid accentua[ting] lines. But blot over to mop up shine and [set] it. You can apply concealer under or over y[our] foundation, blending away edges.

70

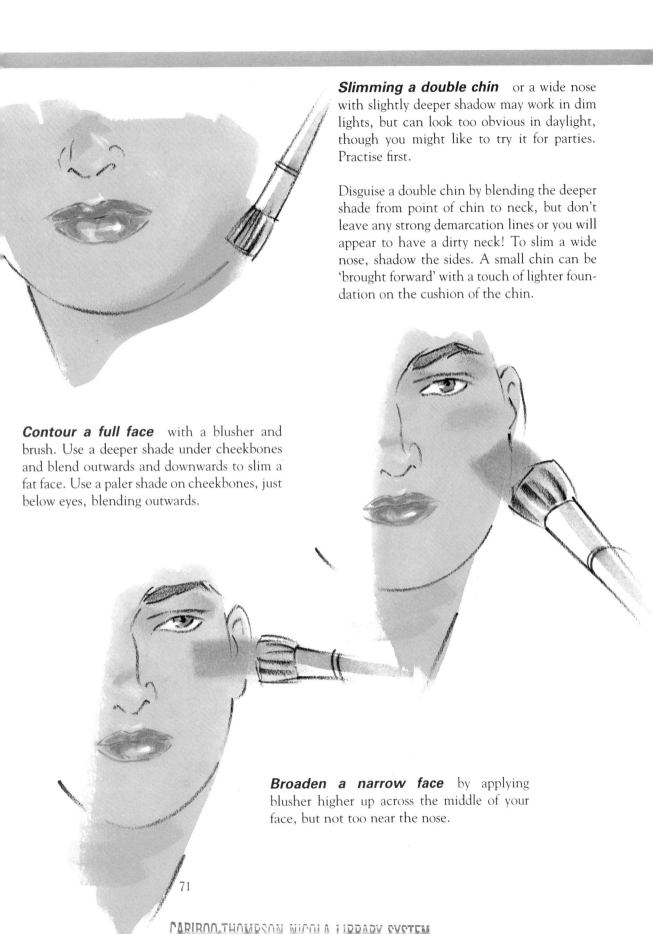

Slimming a double chin or a wide nose with slightly deeper shadow may work in dim lights, but can look too obvious in daylight, though you might like to try it for parties. Practise first.

Disguise a double chin by blending the deeper shade from point of chin to neck, but don't leave any strong demarcation lines or you will appear to have a dirty neck! To slim a wide nose, shadow the sides. A small chin can be 'brought forward' with a touch of lighter foundation on the cushion of the chin.

Contour a full face with a blusher and brush. Use a deeper shade under cheekbones and blend outwards and downwards to slim a fat face. Use a paler shade on cheekbones, just below eyes, blending outwards.

Broaden a narrow face by applying blusher higher up across the middle of your face, but not too near the nose.

CHAPTER 7

A SHOW OF HANDS

Hands get so much wear and tear that it's no wonder they can look rough and age so quickly. In fact, hands are the first give-away of your age, showing up years of sun damage and detergent dryness long before your face, and unlike your complexion, they cannot be disguised with cosmetics. Since the hands have very few oil glands and are frequently exposed to the elements, they become drier faster than any other part of the body, and therefore need consistent moisturizing.

Soap and water damage can cause dermatitis. To prevent this, wear rubber gloves, preferably with thin cotton liners, for wet or dirty chores. While moisturizing hand cream helps to smooth hands temporarily – you have to keep applying them – there are no successful long-term ways to make hands look young. Fat transferral, when cosmetic surgeons use fat suction to take fat from one part of the body (say the bottom of the back) and then inject it into the hands, is not likely to be lasting.

Brown spots, 'liver spots' or age spots are really caused by sunlight. The best way to prevent them is to use a sunscreen all the time.

How to have better nails

The best looking nails have strength and flexibility. Like hair, nails are primarily composed of keratin, a fibrous, porous protein whose cells stretch when nails are exposed to water. The ideal water content for nails is about 16 to 18 per cent. When there is an increase, because of constant wetting, the nails become soft and opaque. But decreased levels of moisture because of using household chemicals and polish removers, and the constant swelling and shrinking of the keratin cells, weaken the bonds that hold together the nail matrix, causing brittleness and dryness.

Tiny dents, cracks and white spots on the nails are caused by injury to the nail matrix. Among the most sensitive areas are the nail bed, under the cuticle, and the lunala, the pale, crescent-shaped portion at the bottom of the nail, where keratin is manufactured. Damage can take from two to six months to surface.

Eating or drinking gelatin in order to try and harden the nails is a waste of time. Nails cannot absorb the protein in gelatin. If you want harder nails, try a nail glaze with hardening agents to form a tough coat that helps protect nails from chipping and breaking.

The average rate of growth in adults is about 0.1 mm per day. Complete regeneration takes about 170 days – for the nail to grow from the lunala to its free edge. But it takes three months before it reaches the lunala. Toenails take longer.

Nails are lifeless in the same way as hair – i.e. there is no blood circulation and they do not contain nerves. However, the nail matrix, the 'womb' of the nail where it is actually produced, is richly supplied with blood capillaries and nerve endings.

The half moon, or lunala, separates the living nail, below the cuticle, from the dead nail which is on view. The cuticle is situated below the half moon and is the epidermis or superficial skin dividing the nail from the rest of the finger. Nails themselves are made up of several layers of dead tissue, held together by particles of oil and moisture to keep them supple and resilient.

Nails vary in thickness from person to person. The rate of growth is not the same for all fingers – the longer the finger, the faster the nail growth.

To stop biting your nails, apply a bitter preparation, or even try false nails.

Nail disorders

Brittleness: As a nail takes six to nine months to grow, if illness has caused the nail to become brittle, it will not appear until about six months after the illness first occurred. Often healthy people complain of brittle nails but you may need to look back six to nine months to find the cause. Anaemia can lead to brittleness but iron medication helps both complaints. Soap and water is the most common cause of brittle nails. It is advisable to wear gloves for all wet work in the house.

Fragile nails: Sometimes nails are influenced by the condition of the nail bed, which in turn is dependent on the blood supply. Disorders of the thyroid and gout have been reported to cause nails to become dry and split. 'Eggshell' nails are when the nail plate becomes soft and semi-transparent, bends easily and splits at the ends. This condition has been associated with arthritis and neuritis (inflammation of a nerve).

The best manicure

When manicuring, hands should not be soaked in soapy water first, as some salon manicurists believe, because soap and water is one of the causes of brittle nails. But you can scrub nails gently with a brush if they need it. Don't use too harsh a nail brush or dig deep down in the pink part of the nail with an orange stick.

If dirt has been pushed down it is best to let it grow out, so that the line dividing the nail tip and the underneath pink part is not pushed down too low. Remove old nail varnish with acetone-free remover. Soak the pad and press against the nail for a moment to dissolve the enamel before wiping off with a few strokes working from base to tip.

Shape nails using an emery board. File in one direction only, not sea-sawing from side to side. Aim to create a rounded tip. It is better not to grow your nails too long because then they are more likely to break and talons can be off-putting.

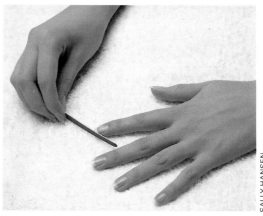

SALLY HANSEN

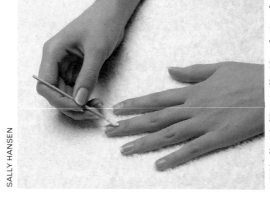

SALLY HANSEN

Never cut your cuticles. They are there to protect the living part of the nail. The correct way to care for them is to keep them supple with creams, then simply push them back gently with cotton wool wrapped round an orange stick, a cotton bud or a rubber-tipped hoof stick. Don't prod too hard.

Swab the nails with a little remover before applying polish. If the nails are greasy, polish won't adhere well. Nails should be clean and dry before you start applying polish.

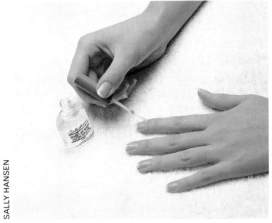

Always use a base coat before you apply the colour – it protects your nails and will give a longer lasting finish. Once your base coat is perfectly dry, apply a first coat of nail varnish as thinly as possible. Follow this with a second thin coat.

After nail varnish is thoroughly dry, give hands a massage with hand cream, and rub cream round the cuticles each evening if you have problem nails.

Nail polish can help to protect your nails – forming a physical barrier and helping them to resist breaking by slowing down the evaporation of water.

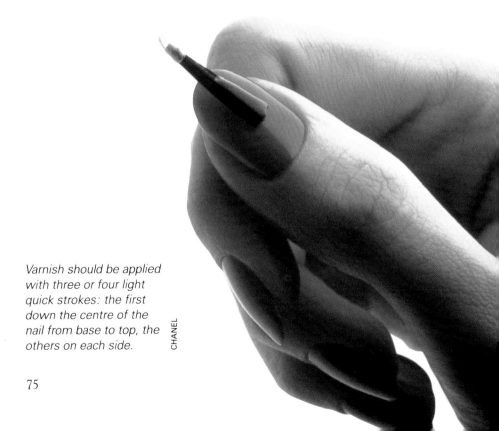

Varnish should be applied with three or four light quick strokes: the first down the centre of the nail from base to top, the others on each side.

75

If you wear polish non-stop, your nails may become less able to regulate the amount of water they retain. Varnish removers are extremely drying, so if your nails keep chipping, it is better to touch-up rather than re-do from scratch, if you can get away with it. Your best bet is to save polish for the occasion rather than using it every day. Pale and clear varnishes don't show the chips as much as deeper colours which can also sometimes stain nails if used for long periods.

CHAPTER 8

ON YOUR FEET

Leonardo da Vinci saw the foot as a work of art and a masterpiece of engineering. That it may be, but for most of us, feet are best kept out of sight and we only tend to think about them when they give us pain and problems.

The foundation of the whole body, feet contain 26 bones, 19 muscles, about 115 ligaments and an intricate network of blood vessels and nerves. Your feet can be adaptable and pliable or they can act as rigid levers. When you walk forward on a flat surface, your body weight is transmitted ideally from your heel, along the outer border and onto the ball of the foot, from where you 'push off' to gain propulsion.

Badly fitting shoes can damage the foot's message systems by working against normal movement, say physiotherapists. Feet are the body's shock absorbers, sustaining a gravity-induced pressure of up to three times your body weight when walking, 10 times when running. But standing seems to be even harder on your feet than moving around, and a foot problem can have effects elsewhere in your body, sometimes throwing out your whole musculo-skeletal alignment.

Most people are born with trouble-free feet, yet two out of five people in a *Which?* magazine survey had suffered a foot problem in the past six months. What turns pretty baby feet into misshapen adult feet? The answer lies inevitably with our shoes.

Spaces between the bones of the child's foot are made up of soft cartilage, which can be moulded by pressure, without pain, so we are not really aware of it. As we grow up, the cartilage 'ossifies' – it is gradually replaced by bone.

If it ossifies into the wrong shape because of badly fitting shoes, or because of an inherited tendency, the foot may end up deformed in some way. Whether or not your feet have emerged from childhood in good shape, what you wear as an adult matters.

Women are twice as likely as men to have foot problems in later years because of not wearing 'foot-worthy' shoes. A lifetime's devotion to fashion will inevitably show up in the shape of your feet.

A foot-worthy shoe . . .

* has a heel no higher than 1 1/2 inch. If the foot is held in place with a strap or laces, even a heel up to 2 1/2 inches may be acceptable, if not for every day. It is best to save high fashion shoes for special occasions – and that goes for slip-ons (even if they are flat, because they do not hold the foot in place) and pointed toes, too. The higher you go, the more your foot is cramped forward into the toes of the shoes.

* fits snugly around the heel so your foot is kept in position. It does not slip up and down.

* is deep enough in the front, so the uppers do not press onto your toes but your feet are held in place, and you can wriggle your toes. Shallow fronted slip-ons make your toes claw to keep them on.

* is 1/4 inch longer than your foot when standing and wide enough to allow your toes to lie naturally, without forcing them to the side, or bunching them together.

* is flexible enough to give you a springy step. It should be supple, where the toe joints bend, but firm in the arch.

Pamper with a pedicure

Cut your toe-nails after the bath while the nails are softened. Remember to cut nails straight across and smooth off the edges with an emery board, but don't have them too short. Don't file down too far at the corners.

Apply an exfoliating foot cream to remove dead skin around the heels and soles. These kind of rough-skin removers contain gritty granules. Or scrub gently with a pumice stone. Don't be too vigorous. You can also remove hard skin with a foot file which has fine and coarse sides.

Clean underneath nails with cotton wool wrapped round an orange stick. Massage cuticle cream into each nail and gently loosen and push back cuticles with a rubber-tipped hoof stick or cotton bud. You can use a cuticle remover cream or lotion if cuticles are sticking to the nailplate. Ease the cuticle back but do not cut or poke too hard.

Give yourself a pedicure after your bath – nails are softer and easier to cut, and cuticles can be gently pushed down more easily.

Massage cream into your feet, then wipe away traces of grease from your toe-nails using a pad soaked in nail varnish remover. This will give a better surface for the varnish to adhere to. Apply a clear base coat as a ridge filler, then two coats of varnish, allowing time to dry. Separate the toes to stop smudging with cotton wool or rubber wedges. Paint on a final transparent top coat to help prevent chipping.

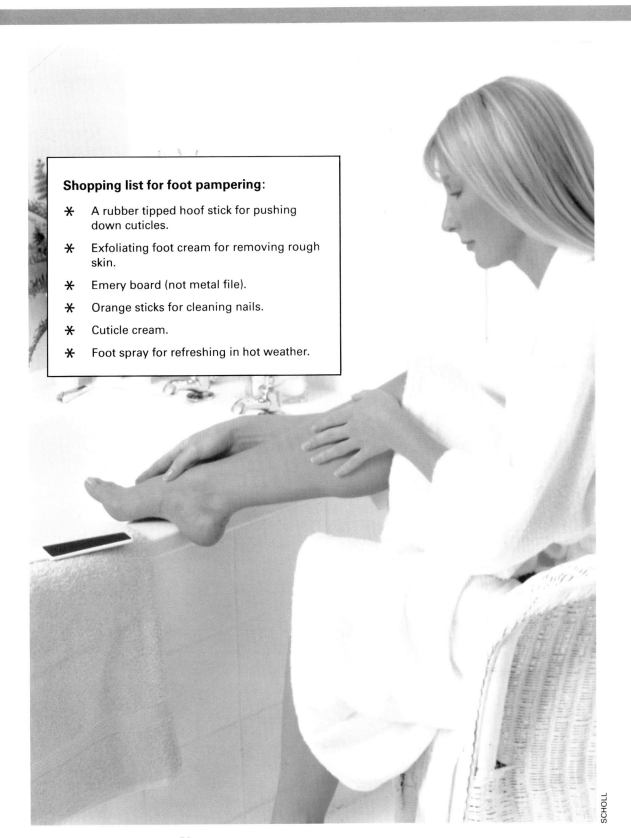

Shopping list for foot pampering:

* A rubber tipped hoof stick for pushing down cuticles.

* Exfoliating foot cream for removing rough skin.

* Emery board (not metal file).

* Orange sticks for cleaning nails.

* Cuticle cream.

* Foot spray for refreshing in hot weather.

SCHOLL

Foot disorders

Hard skin, corns and calluses are the most common foot complaints. Corns are made up of cone-shaped layers of hard dead skin with the pointed end, called the nucleus, facing inwards, causing pain when it presses on a nerve. Hard corns develop on the tips of the toes, and soft corns are found in between the toes.

You can relieve pressure on the corn temporarily, using foam, moleskin or animal wool remedies, available from chemists. But do not attempt to cut or shave off a corn yourself, and corn plasters, which are made with a medicated disc soaked in salicylic acid solution, are not such a good idea because they can injure skin around the corn, too. Best see a chiropodist. Remember, if you don't treat the cause (usually your shoes) then the corn will return.

Calluses are also made of dead hardened skin, caused by shoe friction. It is the skin's protection against irritation, caused probably by the shoe being too wide at the heel and letting the foot slip forward and rub with each step.

You can remove small areas of callus with a special foot file or hard skin pumice stone. Afterwards, massage in an emollient foot cream.

Bunions: one in seven women aged 65 or over in the *Which?* survey had bunions – a problem caused when the fluid cushion around the big toe joint becomes inflamed and thickened. They may be an inherited tendency or caused by ill-fitting shoes worn since childhood. A tendency to have bunions runs in families. Well-fitting shoes can slow down a bunion's development. If they are swollen and painful, see a chiropodist. You may need padding and strapping, and severe cases may be referred for surgery.

Ingrown toe-nails are caused by poorly fitting shoes and by cutting the nails incorrectly. Inevitably it is the big toe-nail that becomes painful and inflamed, with the side of the nail digging into the flesh. Cut toe-nails straight across and just smooth the edges with an emery board to get rid of any roughness. Do not cut nails too short or round them down into the sides. A bad case needs the help of a chiropodist.

Athlete's foot is a fungal infection which grows in moisture and warmth. Synthetic shoes and socks can make the feet perspire and the condition gets worse. Use a special fungicide ointment or solution to clear the condition. You may need to dust your shoes, stockings or socks with athlete's foot powder. Dry carefully between the toes when you bathe.

Verrucas is a viral infection, a foot wart, and should be treated by a chiropodist or your GP. The warts are contagious, and can be caught or passed on to others, for example at public swimming baths.

Smelly feet: there are many sweat glands on the feet, so they will naturally tend to produce an abundance of perspiration. Bacteria ferments the fatty acids found in sweat, so you need to be particularly careful about personal hygiene. Feet need frequent washing and change socks and tights daily. Try to wear cotton socks rather than nylon, and buy all-leather shoes.

Avoid sports shoes with plastic linings or too much nylon in the uppers. Keep an anti-perspirant/deodorant footspray handy. Let your sports shoes dry out – don't keep them in a plastic carrier bag between games.

Chilblains are caused by poor circulation when feet are allowed to become very cold, then subjected to heat, such as a hot water bottle or being close to a fire. Help your feet to retain their natural warmth by wearing warmly lined thick-soled boots in winter – use thermal insoles if there is enough room.

Allow your chilled feet to warm up gradually and massage them with a body lotion or footbalm. Foot exercises can be helpful in stimulating the circulation.

Blisters are caused by your shoes rubbing against tender skin. Cover the pressure point but never pierce the blister. If it breaks spontaneously, wash it with an antiseptic solution and cover with a sterile dressing during the day. At night, leave it uncovered to promote swifter healing.

Heel pain can be caused by heel spurs on the underside of the heel, around a torn or irritated ligament. It is common in athletes but also over-50s can get it when the natural padding on the bottom of the foot starts to wear thin and the heel bone takes most of the pressure when the foot strikes the ground when walking.

Insoles and heel cushions may help. Try to stay off the affected foot as much as you can. Your doctor may give you an injection for immediate relief of pain. Do tendon-stretching exercises before jogging or dancing.

Cramps in your feet and legs may be caused by taking more exercise than usual, or even an abrupt change in heel height up or down, or badly fitting shoes. Try to lift your toes forward to relieve the cramp. Apply a cold damp facecloth.

For suppleness and strength

1. Sit, holding one foot in your hands. One hand holds the heel steady, while the other grasps across the ball of the foot. Keeping your foot quite relaxed, twist the forefoot round in circles, keeping your heel as still as possible. Do 10 times twice daily with each foot.

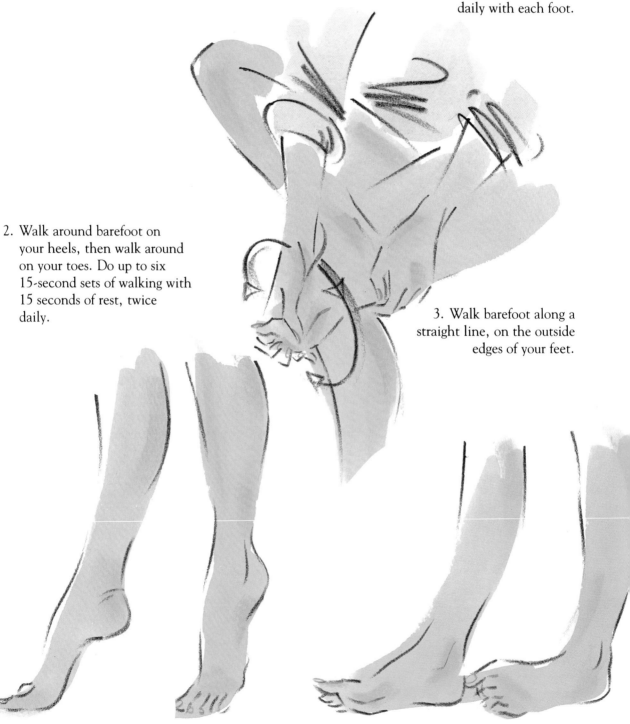

2. Walk around barefoot on your heels, then walk around on your toes. Do up to six 15-second sets of walking with 15 seconds of rest, twice daily.

3. Walk barefoot along a straight line, on the outside edges of your feet.

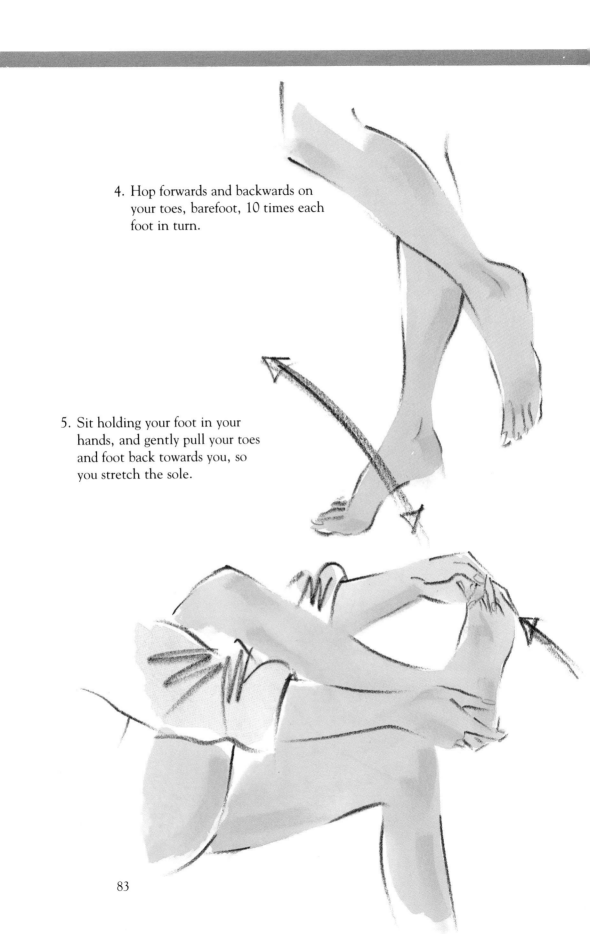

4. Hop forwards and backwards on your toes, barefoot, 10 times each foot in turn.

5. Sit holding your foot in your hands, and gently pull your toes and foot back towards you, so you stretch the sole.

If the shoe fits . . .

Pointed toes and stiletto heels, those prisoners of feet, cramp bones, distort the joints and throw your weight forward onto the metatarsal arch of the foot. The high heel changes your whole anatomy, producing 'a courtship strut', undoubtedly sexy, but imposing strain, and so should be worn for short periods.

Buying shoes by size alone can be misleading, because you may need slightly larger or smaller depending on the manufacturer's lasts and the style.

When buying shoes, stand on tiptoe to see if the heel slides off too easily. Watch for gaps at the sides or too shallow fronts and forget about 'breaking in' shoes eventually. All you will succeed in doing is breaking in your feet.

Varying the height of the heels each day will help to prevent aches and pains – your achilles tendon will adapt to heels worn consistently after a time. Alternating heel heights keeps it flexible.

CHAPTER 9

NECK'S TIME

A woman's age is given away by the condition of her neck and hands long before that of her face, it is said, and it's true. The neck is a part of the body we often neglect or forget and it is a prime target for sun damage. Gravity, tension and fat accumulation also take their toll and the result is wrinkles, jowls, and scraggy skin without elasticity.

The skin on your neck tends to be fine and delicate; it does not have the same amount of sebaceous glands as the skin on the face, and because it is always in the frontline for sun damage, the signs of ageing can show quite early.

Sunlight destroys the collagen and elastic tissue deep in the dermis, a cumulative effect through years of sunbathing, and the neck skin becomes fragile, lined and loose, as if the skin had become bigger than the body it covers.

When you sit in a deckchair or lie down on a beach, it is your neck and the front of the chest which are the prime target for damaging UVA and UVB rays as well as your face. You have only to compare the skin on your neck and chest with that of more protected parts of your body to see the difference.

If you are overweight, the extra fat will no doubt show up round the neck and accumulate round the chinline and it can be the last place to lose fat when you diet. It has been estimated that slimmers need to shed at least 20 lbs before the fat round the neck will be affected.

Poor posture doesn't help. If you walk with your head slumped forward and your chin practically resting on your chest, you are bound to show up double chins even more.

The soft tissues underlying the bony framework of the face and neck are made up of three layers, each susceptible to the effects of age. The deepest layer consists of a complex arrangement of muscles which, because of their contracting power, allow movement of the face and neck.

The thin, large sheet of muscle known as the platysma, suspended from the jaw and extending into the neck, functions as a support, like a built-in chinstrap, and it is this which gives younger people a taut, flat chinline and a well-defined angle at the junction of the neck and jaw. As this muscle ages and loses its tone, however, gravity takes its toll and pulls the flesh out of shape, making it bulge downwards in the form of a jowl and blurring the normal angle between jaw and neck.

When there is more loss of tone, you get vertical ridges of muscle, which overhung by slackened skin, produce folds like a turkey. The upper layer of skin becomes aged prematurely by prolonged exposure to sunlight which destroys the collagen and elastic tissue which support the skin and give it structure. Your skin will gradually lose its firmness and elasticity – pinch a piece of skin and it will not ping back quickly as it does in youth – and creaselines become fixed in the form of grooves or wrinkles.

The third layer, sandwiched between muscle and skin, is the fat and although in youth this is uniformly distributed over the central and lower thirds of the face, it tends to shift down into the neck and jaw, emphasizing the jowl, as we get older.

There are 25 billion fat cells in the body, under the skin, each one filled with a liquid fat, a sticky substance called triglycerides. Fat cells swell up like little balloons but shrink when you diet – they can swell up to three times their size without bursting, and if the body needs to store still more fat, the cells divide to create new ones.

Alas, fat cells put on in middle age are the hardest to get rid of – especially round the chinline. Two chins may be too much but you don't need to be fat or old to get them – it could be because of the shape of your face and jawline, which you inherited.

Beauty care

Impeccably dressed hair for evening glamour: off the face styles show up your bone structure and your neck. Crepey skin and lines can come prematurely when neck skin gets too much sun. Best disguise is a cover-up: a high neck or a choker or a floaty scarf.

Include your neck in all your face and body beauty care but avoid rough stuff, such as exfoliation. If you cleanse your face with lotions and tonics or use a rinsable cleanser or soap, don't forget your neck, too. But most importantly, do moisturize it morning and night as you do your face.

Special neck creams are generally made up of a heavier and richer formula because the skin of the neck tends to be dry and rather less sensitive than the face. But you don't need to get a special cream just for your neck – your face creams will do. Massage in creams starting at the base of the neck and

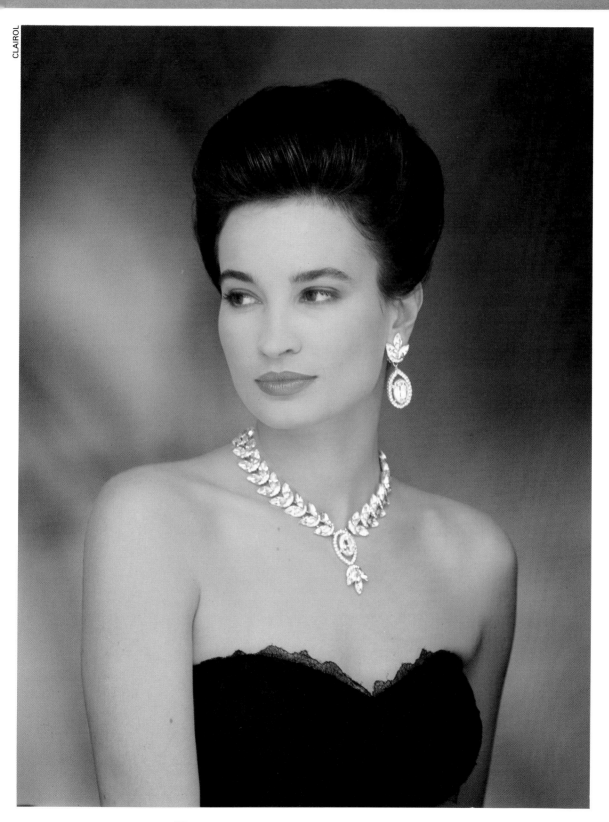

working upwards with hand-over-hand movements. Use the outside of the hands to smooth the cream under the chin and towards the ears.

Even if you have neglected your neck in the past, you can begin afresh today, and above all, protect it from sunlight. Use a highly protective sunscreen – the higher the better – and reapply it frequently through the day when on holiday.

You can use a moisturizer which contains sun filters, too. If you want to sunbathe, keep a scarf handy to cover your neck and the front of your chest if you want to stop any more signs of ageing.

Cosmetic surgery

The neck lift (another name for the face-lift) is the only way to restructure the jawline permanently. The operation involves the lifting and tightening of the under-jaw muscle, removal of excess fat with fat suction, and the partial excision and remodelling of the facial skin. It is a major operation. See chapter 10 for more details.

Disguise tactics

If you can't change it, you can always disguise it. Soft scarves and collars help to camouflage a crêpey neck. So does a hairstyle with soft, casual waves or a bob that covers the point where jaw meets neck. An off-the-face style or very short hair can throw unwanted attention on the neck.

On the other hand, if your skin can stand the spotlight, a short neck can be made to appear longer with a short upswept hairstyle. Longer hair left hanging tends to swamp. A V-neck or open shirt collar can make a neck seem longer, whereas a roll-neck or high collar tends to shorten.

Cosmetic camouflage techniques with make-up are never very successful because the shading can make you look as though you had a dirty neck in daylight. Save such theatrical tricks for dim lighting. Then you can try a little shading with a touch of browny blusher under the chin from ear to ear, blending in well. You can add a touch of highlight to the pad of a small chin to 'bring it forward'.

Neck savers

To try to prevent fat settling round your neck and jawline, you obviously need to watch your weight, and in particular, watch your fat

Neck skin soon shows your age. Always apply the skin cream you use on your face onto the neck, and protect it carefully from collagen-destroying sunlight.

HELENA RUBINSTEIN

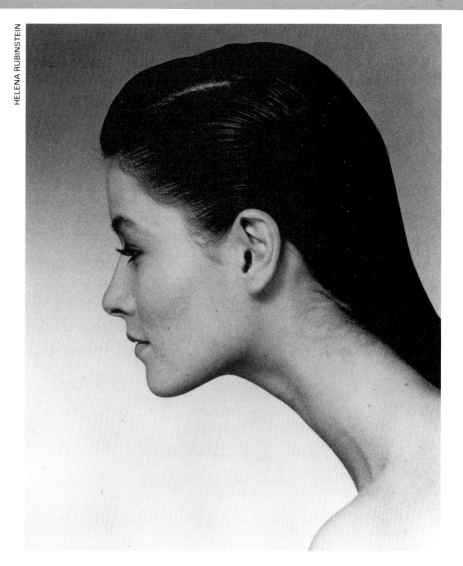

intake (See Slim tips, page 122). If you need to lose weight, don't try to do it quickly. It is much better for your body and your health to lose excess weight slowly, no more than a pound a week, eating a healthy, varied diet. Older people who lose a lot of weight quickly find it tends to leave the neck wrinkled and scraggy-looking.

To ease neck tension . . .   try giving yourself a neck massage. Place your hands each side of the neck at the back with thumbs round the front. Starting at your shoulder blades as far down as you can comfortably reach, and keeping fingers together, stroke firmly upwards. Knead the base of the neck at the back. Clasp one hand over the other and press heels of hands firmly onto the neck on either side at the back. Press and release as you move hands up and down the neck.

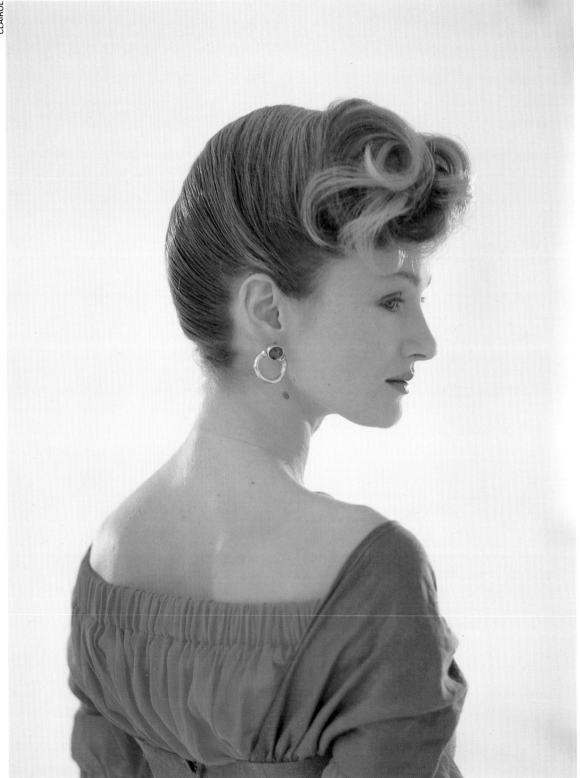

CHAPTER 10

BEYOND THE FRINGE

Your hair says a lot about you without you even needing to say a word. It can make you look dated or up-to-the-minute, staid or wild, formal or casual. Seat of the soul, symbol of strength or pure decoration, hair may be dead the moment it leaves the scalp but it has a very live part to play in our self-esteem and how others perceive us and our personality. Above all, your hair is your most important beauty accessory and with it, you can add or subtract the years.

Young hair looks smooth and shiny, not over-processed and dull. When we are young, it is virgin hair, untouched by chemicals and mechanical aids. But once we start on the tinting or perming path, and use electrically heated hairstylers, all to often the result can be dry, lack-lustre locks, without shine or elasticity.

There are over 100,000 hairs on the average head and we spend a lot of time,s money and effort trying to make them look good. But all too often things go wrong. Not that you can just sit back and do nothing, of course. But you need to treat your hair literally as your crowning glory and give it the care and respect you would give to, say an expensive cashmere sweater.

What is hair made of?

To look after your hair in the best possible way, it pays to know something of its composition and how our hair products affect it.

Hair is a form of protein, known as keratin, which is a similar material to that of our finger and toe-nails. Each hair grows out of a follicle or dip in the scalp (otherwise known as a pore), with cells forming and dividing at the very base of each hair follicle, and being fed nutrients by the blood.

Beautifully 'dressed' hair by Richard Dalton of Claridges shows off smooth skin and a firm jawline. Once the outline gets blurred you may want to try styles that offer more 'foliage' cover.

There is a period of growth and a period of rest before each hair falls out and a new hair grows to replace it. During the growth (anagen) phase, the hair will grow about half an inch a month and this phase lasts up to six years. If your hair doesn't grow very long naturally, it could be because you have a shorter anagen phase. The resting phase (telogen) is about three months and this is when the hair is shed. Normally about 85 per cent of hair is in the growth phase and 15 per cent is resting.

91

If you could see a single hair under the microscope, you would find that it is divided into three basic layers. The outer cuticle is made up of tiny overlapping scales, like the tiles on a roof. Underneath is a cortex layer, where the pigment is stored, and in the middle, a medulla core, although this is absent in very fine hair.

The appearance of your hair is affected by the state of the scales on the outer layer of hair. When hair is in good condition, the little scales lie flat and close together, the hair feels silky and light is reflected giving the shine we all seek.

But when the hair is dry or damaged, the cuticle scales lift, curl at the edges and separate, your hair will tangle easily, feel dull and porous and light reflection will be poor. Raised scales also mean that the protective armour that surrounds each hair is bridged, which leaves the vulnerable inner hair exposed.

The cortex within is made up of long bundles of cells held in place by bonds or links – these can be broken by water and temporarily reformed into a curl shape when styled with a brush or roller and dried. But as soon as the hair absorbs moisture again, the bonds revert back to their original pattern. The chemicals in perms rearrange the cells and bonds permanently.

A strand of hair can be as personal as a fingerprint. It is possible to detect through laboratory tests your blood group, sex, approximate age and even whether you have taken drugs.

Although stress and pressure may affect hair in the long run – as well as the rest of your body – it is mechanical abuse of hair because of styling equipment and hair processing chemicals that cause most hair damage. Anything that applies heat directly to the hair causes some damage and it is a matter of how little damage you can get away with.

LIMITING THE DAMAGE

Dry hair

Our hair becomes dry usually because of what we have been doing to it. It is true that our sebaceous glands tend to produce less oil as we get older – teenage greasy locks and skin become less greasy with the passing years, but hair is basically dry because of self-inflicted damage.

Chemicals used in perms, bleaches and permanent colourants lift the scales on the hair shaft in order to penetrate into the cortex layer beneath, and they are not fully smoothed down again afterwards, leaving a tendency to dryness and porosity. The more chemicals you use on your hair, the more the inevitable dryness and damage: it becomes over-processed. The hair becomes weakened, less elastic and may break, and there will be loss of shine. Sunlight, too, tends to dry the hair, as does regular use of heated hair stylers and dryers, and electrically heated rollers.

In theory, the oils secreted by the sebaceous glands on the scalp should be distributed down the length of the hair with brushing. Years ago, brushing with a bristle brush was part of every woman's beauty routine. But how many of us brush our hair today? Too much brushing can also break and split the hair, that's true, but used judiciously, a good bristle brush can still be beneficial.

But what if you have a perm or curly hair, or the type of hair that seems impossible to brush because of style or thickness? Use a brush-styler with wide-apart filaments to distribute your conditioner after you shampoo.

We wash our hair much more often these days. Years ago, it was probably once a week. Now it is more like three times a week, and young people with short hair may wash it every day. This, too, can contribute to dryness because although you may use a mild, frequent-wash shampoo, you are still removing a certain percentage of the hair's natural oils.

It's a hair-raising thought, but a survey has discovered that more than eight million women in Britain today share exactly the same hair problem: coping with dry, splitting ends. Dry ends are a drag because, left untreated, the split will travel up the hair shaft and get steadily worse. The hair looks wispy, perhaps frizzy and out of sorts, and you will find it difficult to style.

The cure is to reach for the scissors – or rather to ask your hairdresser to give you a trim. Split ends need cutting off. An intensive all-over conditioner smoothes the hair cuticles and makes hair easier to comb, so there's less chance of damage. If the hair nearest the scalp tends towards oiliness, apply the conditioner directly just to the hair ends after shampooing and towel-drying.

Use one application of shampoo, not two. That is not necessary when you wash your hair a lot. Blot hair with a towel and don't rub hard. As wet hair tends to stretch and may break (wet hair stretches up to 30 per cent of its length and weak hair snaps, like old elastic), comb through your hair carefully using a good quality wide-toothed comb or brush-styles, with rounded ended teeth or filaments.

Try not to do too much heat-styling. Heat raises the scales allowing the hair's natural moisture to escape. Before using dryers, tongs, rollers or stylers, it is a good idea to condition your hair well after shampooing, because this will help replace lost moisture and close the cuticle, sealing in moisture and protecting the cortex within.

It is better to let hair dry naturally and avoid using spiky brushes, combs, and rubber bands. Always cover up hair as much as possible in hot sunlight, especially if you have been using colourants or perms.

Dry hair needs to be conditioned every time you wash it and if you have time, use a thicker cream treatment that is left on the hair for about 20 minutes before rinsing. Some conditioners are meant to be left on and not rinsed off.

In between shampoos, use spray-on hair shiners and hair dressings, particularly if hair is thick, coarse and curly as well as dry. The occasional warm-oil conditioning treatment can be a useful addition to your beauty care routine, especially after a holiday. You can buy an oil treatment or make your own using almond oil . . . any oil will probably do, but you may not like the smell. Warm the oil by standing a cup in hot water and apply to the hair, massaging in well. Cover your head with a bath cap and a warm towel and shampoo off after about an hour.

Weathering the damage

Heated styling brushes are a boon for giving curl, direction and volume and helping to control frizzy bits.

Your environment can affect the condition of your hair, too. Central heating and air conditioning have a drying effect on both hair and skin, reducing moisture levels. Outside, wind, cold, sun and sea all play their part. Add the salt from the sea and chlorine from pools and you have all the ingredients of a Molotov cocktail that will not do you any good.

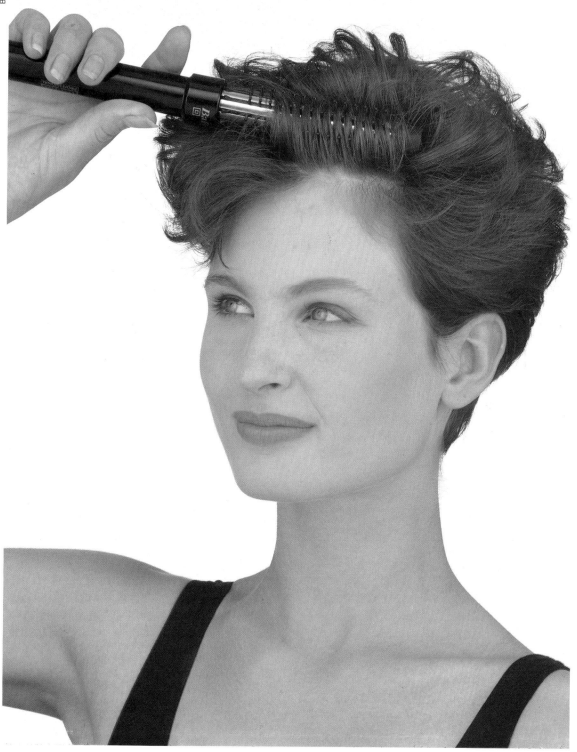

Use gentle shampoos on holiday and take plenty of conditioner. Always rinse your hair well after bathing in either sea or pool and use a conditioner before you comb it through. Sunlight will tend to strip the colour from coloured or bleached hair, increasing porosity. So it might be worth trying hair products that contain sun filtering ingredients as well as conditioners.

How to cope with over-processed hair

Given that you want to continue with permanent tinting (if you are going grey) or to have perms, you will have to treat your hair with care, choosing shampoos, conditioners and styling aids especially formulated for damaged or tinted and processed hair. Conditioning helps elasticity and strength and encourages the cuticle scales to lie flat and close together, giving extra shine and body.

Kinder colour? If you have been bleaching your hair for some time, you will find that retouching the roots without overlapping already treated hair is not easy to do. It is more expertly dealt with by a salon, but damage can still occur. Full-head bleaching done regularly is probably the most damaging thing that you can do to your hair, so to regain hair strength and lustre, consider highlights instead as an alternative. This way, you won't have to keep retouching the roots so often, and you can leave it much longer between colouring sessions. Your hairdresser may advise you to have lowlights put in the blonde to get your highlights off to a good start.

Covering grey? Go for natural tones rather than stronger tints. If you used to be brunette, a shade or two lighter than your original hair colour can be more flattering.

CLAIROL

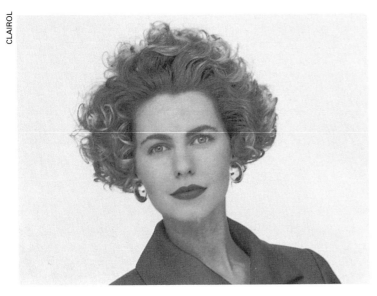

If you have regular permanent tints to cover grey and your root regrowth begins to show after about three weeks, consider having a hairstyle that is more root camouflaging, and then you can leave longer intervals between tints. Smooth, close-to-the-head styles with partings tend to show your roots quickly, while styles that have body, which are curly and wavy, are more disguising.

In between your permanent tint retouching, try using a kinder semi-permanent colour in a similar shade. This just stains the outside of the

96

hair and washes out gradually. As semi-permanents do not contain oxidizing agents, they do not lift the hair scales and cause porosity.

Permanent waving lotions, too, have a drastic effect on the hair and make it very porous and dry. So try to leave longer gaps between perms and look to other curling methods that don't necessitate using chemicals . . . like pipecleaner sets and special setting and styling aids. Before and after every perm, be sure to give your hair plenty of conditioning. Have the ends of your permed hair trimmed regularly to get rid of splits and brittleness and investigate hairstyles that don't need so much perm support.

If your hair is very limp, try firmer gels, extra strength mousses, and firm hold hairsprays for setting and styling. Some sprays can be used on damp or dry hair to hold and moisturize.

Naturally fine hair can take advantage of the new generation of perm lotions, which are called acid waves, keeping hair in a natural acid state during processing and thus avoiding some, if not all, the damage.

Long hair

The longer your hair, the older the ends, and these are particularly vulnerable to wear and tear. Natural oil produced at scalp level is unable to travel down the length of long hair to condition the ends, where it is most needed, so use a natural bristle brush, and apply plenty of conditioner to hair ends when washing.

Even if you are growing your hair, have the ends cut regularly to stop splitting. Tangling can be a problem, too, and conditioning helps to stop you tugging and causing more hair damage.

Fine texture

Fine textured hair is often a flop. It lies close to the scalp, looks greasy quickly, doesn't hold a set for long, and lacks body. So how can you thicken your thatch?

Sometimes, having hair tinted seems to make it a bit more manageable, either highlights or all-over permanent colouring. The hair coarsens up slightly, seeming thicker. A perm is obviously a solution but investigate different types – it may be you just need a root-perm.

Get a good cut and have it trimmed about every three weeks, so it doesn't look ragged. A blunt cut style, where hair is cut straight across, and not thinned out into too many layers, is thought to make thin hair look thicker.

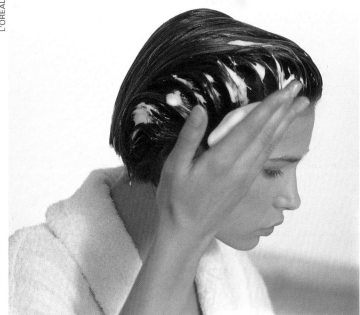

L'ORÉAL

Use hair setters such as gels, mousses and sprays. Blow-dry the hair upside down, scrunching with your hands for more volume, and spray the roots.

Stop hair going flat on top – long hair layers 'drag' hair down because of the weight and make it cling more closely to the scalp. For more fullness on top, you need shorter layers, even though the ends get blunt cut for a thicker effect. Then you can add gel or mousse as a style support. Try setting top hair on hot rollers to get a lift, occasionally, as too much heat styling can be drying.

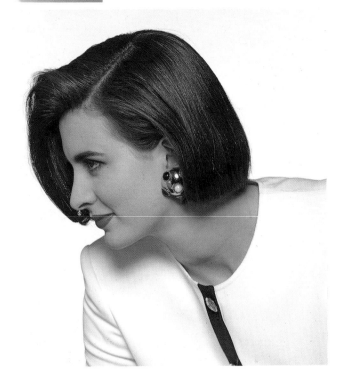

ELIDA GIBBS

Have hair cut to collar-length, no longer. A body perm helps to make hair look thicker because your hair style will have more volume and won't lie so close to the scalp.

Shine on

Long or short, hair is more attractive when it looks glossy and shiny. But what is this elusive quality? Shine is the reflection of light on an object: the smoother the surface, the more direct and intense the reflection. So straight hair is going to have more shine than curly hair, whatever you do to it. The wavy pattern produces an uneven surface so hair is less likely to reflect light.

Besides the degree of straightness or curl, other factors play a part in your hair's glossiness, including density: the more strands you have per square inch of scalp, the better. Thick hair also makes a better reflective surface, whereas light passes right through thin hair.

Conditioners formulated from synthetic polymers instantly smooth uneven hair surfaces for optimum light reflection and deposit a transparent resin which also reflects light. These chemicals form a surface film and bond to the outer hair surface, smoothing and filling in damage, if only temporarily, though protein is thought to have a beneficial effect on breakages.

Hair loss

Normally, we can lose between 70 and 100 hairs a day and not even notice it. Hair is replacing itself all the time. Healthy, luxuriant hair is associated with youth, and thinning hair with ageing, so it is always a worry to find you are losing more hair than you are replacing.

There are four main causes for hair loss: systemic (reaction to drugs and ill health), scalp disease, heredity and mechanical trauma.

In any instance of undue hair loss do go and see your doctor. If you are taking any medication, abnormal thyroid function could be a culprit. Women may find that their hair becomes thinner because of hormonal adjustments and changes: about three to six months after childbirth, for example, though hair usually returns to its original thickness after a while; or after the menopause.

With *alopecia areata*, sudden hair loss, you lose clumps of hair and bald patches form on the scalp. This problem can happen with both men and women, and it has been estimated that as many as one in a hundred people can lose hair through this distressing scalp disease, though it has long been a fairly secret problem as some people may not even see their GP about it.

The causes of the disease are baffling but it is thought to be almost certainly an auto-immune disease in which some of the white blood cells overwork and produce antibodies to attack hair follicles as though they were foreign bodies.

You may lose hair because of shock or illness. *Traction alopecia* is when hair is lost because of tightly pulled pony-tails, braids and chignons, or by hair-tugging. Hair bands, wigs and hats that are too tight can also cause hair to be lost.

Common male pattern baldness is caused by the action of the male sex hormones, the androgens, on hair follicles, and is genetic. Some women, too, may also have the misfortune to get the condition, though they have no other signs of masculinity.

Certain progesterones in the Pill and hormone replacement therapy are suspected of having an influence on hair loss, too. Endocrinologists are now looking more critically at pills which contain 'androgenic progesto-gens' such as norethisterone, ethynodiol diacetate, lynoestronel or nor-gestrel, and doctors find alternatives for patients with hair loss problems.

In severe cases of alopecia, there has been some success in the use of minoxidil, the medication originally discovered as a side-effect of a blood pressure remedy. This is applied to the scalp direct, or used together with retinoic acid (the acne preventative which dermatologists now believe can have a rejuvenating effect on sun-damaged skin). The two together seem to work better than minoxidil on its own.

In any case of hair loss, do see your doctor, who may well refer you to a special hair or dermatology clinic. Happily, a lot of the time hair grows back naturally again.

Grey or not to grey?

Grey hair can creep up on you . . . from the odd white hair to a sprinkling, then a concentration, perhaps, round the hairline. Do you want to fight it or give in gracefully? The age when you start going grey is usually a matter of heredity. Some find they even start greying at 15 but most of us begin to see white hairs in our mid-30s, and a few lucky people can keep their colour later.

If you want to stay grey, semi-permanents can still be useful to get the right sort of tone . . . not too yellow, not too blue.

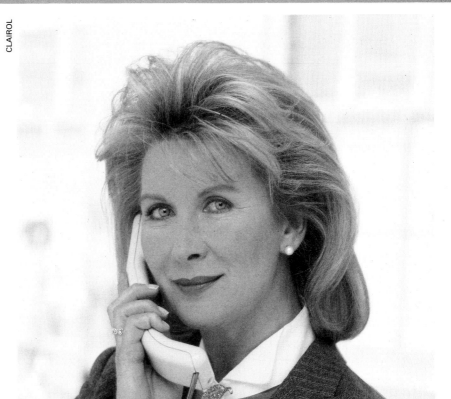

What we call 'grey' hair is really white, or no-colour hair, when pigment is no longer produced in the hair bulb, to be passed on to the hair's cortex layer (see page 92). You can pluck out odd white hairs at first, but there will come a time when you either submit to nature, or fight it.

Hair signifies youth and sexuality, so although there are some of us who look wonderful with grey hair, there is also the feeling that you are unconsciously saying 'goodbye' to all that kind of thing. You may still feel 25 inside, but you may be giving off different kinds of vibes.

How good you look with greying hair also depends on your original hair colour. If you are dark, the result will be pepper-and-salt. If you are a natural blonde, the grey will be hidden for longer. Redheads look faded.

Smoking can make grey hair yellow in front (yet another reason to stop). A toning semi-permanent colourant that washes out over six shampoos can subtly enhance.

The white hairs tend to be coarser and more wiry, so even a scattering can show up in dark hair. If you have a young, unlined skin, then silver hair can look dramatic. Blonde hair merges into silver and goes well with a naturally fair skin.

Stay grey?   Silvery hair can look most distinguished but it needs care to prevent it becoming dry, wiry and dull-looking. With the loss of the colouring melanin pigment from the hair, there is often also a loss of moisture and elasticity. White hairs are coarser.

If you smoke, white hair will yellow, particularly in front, though there are products you can buy to prevent discolouration. Semi-permanents in ashy silver or slate shades are enhancing. Colour mousses and colour setting lotions come in pearly hues to tone down yellowness, too. Chose a shampoo and conditioner for dry and damaged hair.

CLAIROL

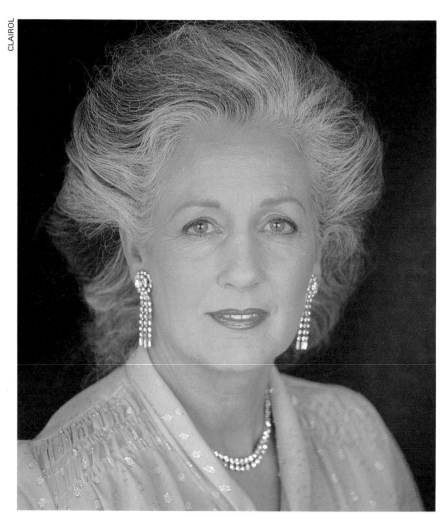

Facing page: Stark white hair can look very dramatic but the texture may seem coarse and dry, so use plenty of conditioner every time you shampoo. Low lights can be threaded through if you want a change.

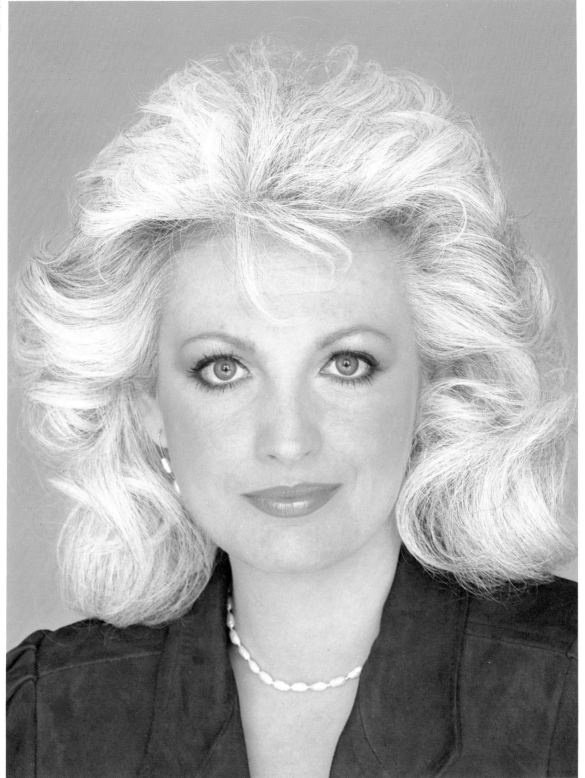

Count on colour After 60, you may decide that you want to look natural, and give in, but many of us want to cling on to colour and that means using colourants. What kind of camouflage colour you choose depends on the percentage of grey in your hair. A more gentle semi-permanent colourant, especially formulated for greying hair, will blend in the white hairs with your original hair shade. Choose a shade closest to your own colour. As semi-permanents just stain the outside of the hair cuticle, they wash out a little every time you shampoo, and you will need to reapply them fairly frequently. On the other hand, these kind of colourants are kind to hair and make it look in good condition.

But if you have around 30 per cent of white hairs, or a concentration of white in one area, you need a stronger effect, achieved with a permanent colourant. These necessitate mixing together two kinds of ingredients – the dye with an oxidizing ingredient – to be able to penetrate the outer hair scales into the cortex beneath.

The more grey you have, the more you should consider going a tone or two lighter than your original hair colour when you were younger. It will look softer and far more natural. And do consider your complexion, too.

Very dark brown or black can accentuate the lines on your face and make you look even older. The dark Latin look hair of 25 should mellow into a medium warm brown at 39, and lighten to a softer brown over 50. If you like to be blonde, go for more subtle, subdued hues, never too gold or platinum, and consider highlights.

Your hair is not just one colour but is composed of several shades all mingling together. So dyeing your hair one dark matt shade can look unnatural and hard.

The trouble with permanents (and don't forget that bleaches are permanent, too, but they subtract colour rather than adding it) is that they can lead to dryness and over-processed hair which lacks elasticity and shine. Grey roots will show through in about three weeks and will need to be retouched. That's the problem you have to face once you start on the dyeing route. The idea is to apply the colourant. to the roots, but not to the already coloured hair – or at least not for long – to stop over-processing.

If you have been covering your grey hair and want to go natural, stop using a permanent colour and switch to a semi-permanent in the same shade. Continue to use this, reapplying after about every five shampoos, until your hair grows out.

You can use semi-permanents at home fairly easily, but when it comes to permanent tints, it is hard to do the roots yourself without overlapping onto already processed hair, unless you have a friend to help, or you are particularly skilful.

Salon colour is obviously more expensive, and the commitment can be considerable with roots growing through. See section on over-processed hair on page 96 for more ideas about how to cope.

A question of style

Even if you have had long hair all your life, consider a cut as you get older – or at least do not wear your hair more than shoulder-length. Long hair can 'drag' the face down, What you need is a frame to the face, softness and some volume. As Colette once said: a face needs foliage.

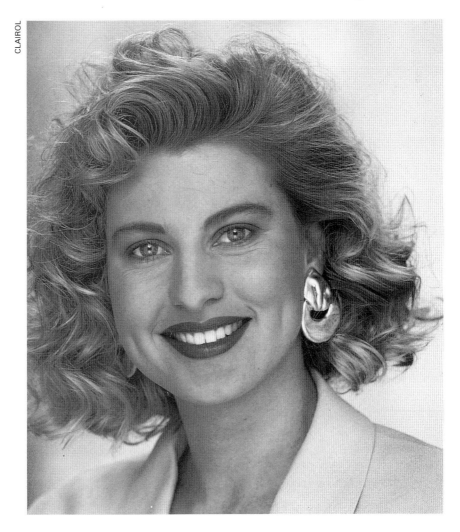

CLAIROL

Soft curls and waves give a face more flattering 'foliage' than starker styles.

A half fringe or bang can soften a style and make it look less hard.

Too short hair can be hard to get away with. There's nothing to hide behind and it can be cruelly revealing of a wrinkled neck and drooping chinline. Some hair over the forehead obviously hides lines and brow furrows. But there are no hard and fast rules. The best way to get a hairstyle that makes you look younger is to find a hairdresser with the skill to create a style that looks good on you.

You can look older when you hang on to a style that looked fine when you were younger, but which has become dated. Hair can be the last thing about herself a woman changes. It takes courage (and faith in your hairdresser) to try a new image.

Have you always worn a severe blunt-cut, chin-length helmet bob? Very stark geometric styles usually look best with young features and it could be you need it slightly softening. Tight curly perms can also look ageing and old fashioned.

Pulling your hair back or up in a bun or chignon may look elegant, but is it now too hard for your features? Very stiff, formal styles may also look matronly. Trying to look too young can be ageing. So avoid bows, bizarre shapes and colours. A kind of planned carelessness can be flattering, with hair that is shiny soft, and which moves.

REVLON

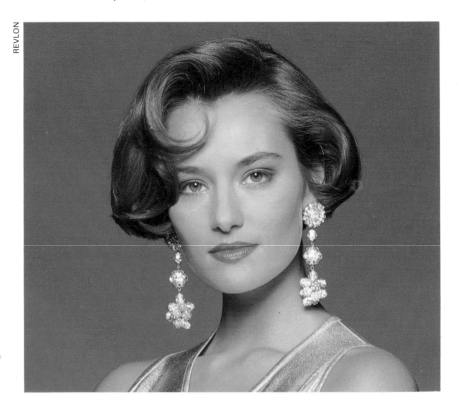

Facing page: Casual short cut is easy on the eye and easy to keep up. Scrunch with fingers and a little mousse for a crisper texture.

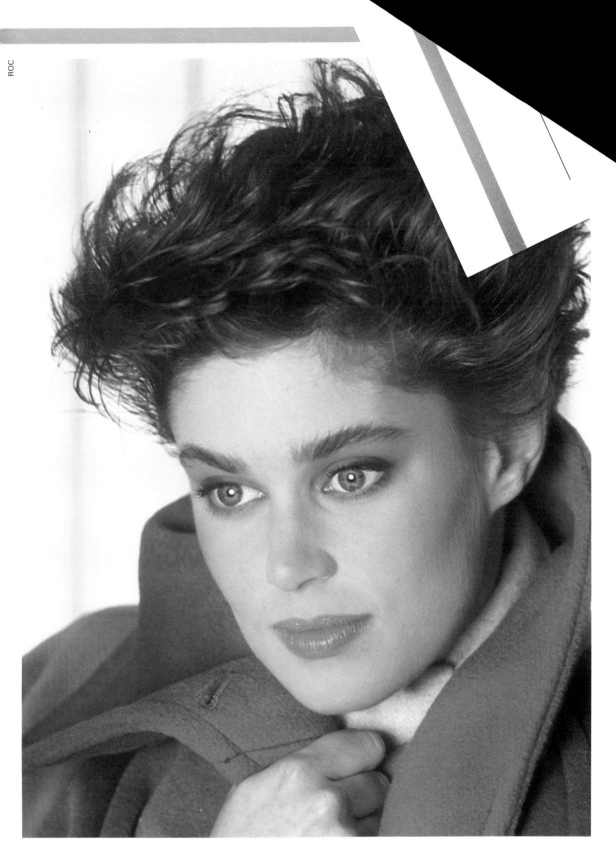

CHAPTER 11

OPERATION BEAUTY

Cosmetic surgery is the most extreme solution to any beauty problem. But before you submit yourself to the scalpel in the search for a redesigned face or body, you should find out all you can about the subject, and be very selective in your choice of surgeon.

There are no more than 150 fully trained plastic surgeons in the UK, and double that number in New York alone. Although in the UK cosmetic surgery is done under the National Health Service, waiting lists are long and priority is given to people with disfigurements and reconstructions as a result of serious illness or accidents.

If you have a physical problem, such as over-large breasts, that is causing you distress, it is worth asking your GP for a referral to a hospital consultar.t plastic surgeon. If he considers you a suitable case for treatment, you will go on the waiting list – the lists vary from hospital to hospital and according to the priority rating assigned to you.

To have surgery done privately, it is still a good idea to ask your GP for a referral to a reputable surgeon, who will no doubt be a consultant in the NHS with a private practice. A personal recommendation is always worth considering. But if you do not know anyone who has had cosmetic surgery, beware of commercial clinics which advertise because there are many cowboys in this field and you do not want to risk being operated on by someone who is not fully qualified or experienced.

The problem with trying to find a suitable surgeon is that the General Medical Council does not allow doctors to advertise and information about qualified surgeons is given only to other doctors. However, if your GP is not sympathetic about your interest in cosmetic surgery, you can find a reputable surgeon by looking up the plastic surgery unit in your local NHS hospital, in the Medical Directory, in your public library. If you ring up the unit secretary, you should be able to find out the private practice number of the NHS consultant plastic surgeon. Any reputable surgeon will write to your own GP as a matter of medical courtesy, to keep him informed.

Most consultant plastic surgeons (who also do cosmetic surgery) will be members of one or both of the two professional associations: the British Association of Plastic Surgeons (BAPS) and the British Association of Aesthetic Plastic Surgeons (BAAPS).

Are your expectations realistic?

You do not have to worry about being thought vain if you go to see a plastic surgeon. Vanity is probably the one sin of which he might approve! If you go in for cosmetic surgery, you should be doing it for yourself, to give yourself more self-confidence perhaps, not because you think it will save a marriage.

Perhaps you have a physical defect that makes you feel so different from other people that you suffer mental distress. Unattractive features can cause misery although they may not be a danger to your health. Psychologically, it may prey on your mind and diminish the quality of your life. But surgeons are careful to screen patients with deep psychological problems, or unrealistic expectations, because such people are never satisfied.

It is not reasonable to try to achieve extreme standards of physical perfection. Whatever the surgeon's skills, all surgery entails risk and you may trade a minor disfigurement for a scar. Nobody can forecast how you will heal.

When you have a consultation with the surgeon (which ideally you will have chosen with the assistance of your GP), you should ask him to say what he thinks he can achieve and what are the shortcomings of any technique. In the light of that, you have to decide whether you can live with the shortcomings.

Touching up

Sometimes one plastic surgery operation can lead to another: you might need a second operation to tidy up the scars from the first, or to make some adjustments. It would be wise to ask the surgeon before your initial operation if you will have to pay more. Some surgeons will always charge for a touch-up procedure – but some do not. However, you will undoubtedly be charged by the anaesthetist and the hospital.

A tummy tuck operation – a complete abdominal reduction – inevitably needs a touch-up to tidy the scars. About 10 per cent of all rhinoplasties do, too, and eye and breast augmentations may also need adjusting.

The lifestyle factor

Your way of life before and after surgery is an important consideration in order to achieve the best results. Smoking, in particular, is linked to poor healing and increased risk of scarring after surgery. Both smoking and drinking spirits can affect bruising.

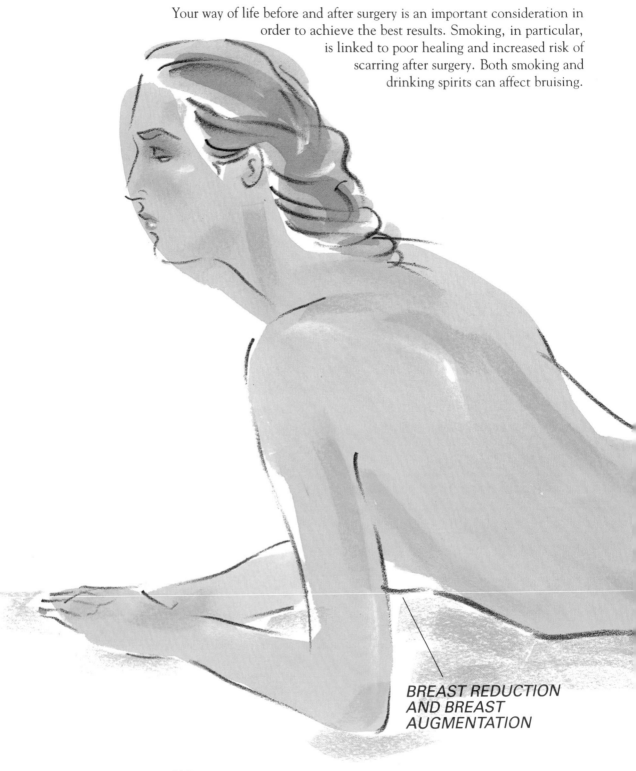

BREAST REDUCTION AND BREAST AUGMENTATION

Smoking leads to bigger problems with anaesthesia after any operation and can give increased swelling round the eyes after a nose reconstruction. It is thought to narrow the capillaries that carry blood to the face, just as it constricts major arteries. After surgery, a smoker's blood vessels may not deliver enough blood to the incision sites.

After a face-lift, surgeons recommend avoiding sport and strenuous activity for four weeks and prolonged exposure to the sun and heat for three months, for example. Whether or not you believe in vitamin C for healing, it might be worth considering taking 1 gm tablets of vitamin C daily for at least two weeks before undergoing surgery, just in case.

THE DESIGNER BODY

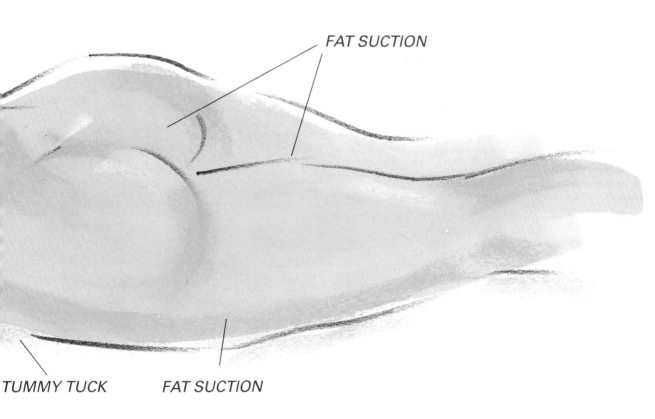

FAT SUCTION

TUMMY TUCK   FAT SUCTION

TREATING SKIN PROBLEMS

Birthmarks

The most common cosmetic surgery operations usually involve the removal of an unwanted skin blemish, such as a birthmark, cyst or nodule. A very obvious skin stain can be extremely stressful and although camouflaging it with a pigmented cover cream can work well, there are now surgical ways in which some stains can be treated.

Port wine stains If you have a port wine stain on your skin you may be referred to a variety of specialists – an opthalmic surgeon, for example, a plastic surgeon or a dermatologist. The stain may cover part of the face, neck, head, even arms and hands, and is caused by a tightly knit network of fine capillary blood vessels.

The newest way to treat some types of blood vessel birthmarks is with a *laser*, and the latest Tunable Dye Laser is particularly useful because it produces a much more precise burn around the blood vessels in the skin than other lasers, and therefore the chances of it altering the skin texture or producing any scarring are very small. Selectively damaging the abnormal blood vessels with a laser results in some skin peeling, crusting and scabbing about a week or ten days later. Very often the whole thing heals without problems.

Usually it is possible to produce some sort of improvement in a port wine stain, but the question is whether that improvement is significant or not and whether it makes any real difference to the camouflage make-up you may need to use, and how you feel about the problem. Diathermy, using burning electric currents, may also be used but if the blood vessels are deep, and do not cover too broad an area, a skin graft may be considered.

A superficial stain can be improved with laser therapy, but there is no completely satisfactory method as yet.

Brown birthmarks are usually superficial, in the topmost layers of the skin, in the first few weeks after a baby is born, and using dermabrasion (surgical planing) to sandpaper away the stain can be extremely successful – although a traumatic idea for the parents to accept.

Moles can be removed quite simply at any time in your life, if they are unsightly, but there will be a scar, hopefully of much lesser importance, which will fade in time.

Tattoos   Getting rid of an unwanted tattoo isn't easy and everything from pigeon's excrement to acids have been used through the ages with sometimes unpleasant results. But today, carbon dioxide and ruby lasers are successfully used to vaporize the ink.

It is not a painless procedure, and more than one treatment may be needed to make sure the pigment is finally removed; and you may be left with pale scars, but if you really hate the tattoo, the laser is probably the most successful means of removal.

Acne scars   'Sandpapering' techniques such as *dermabrasion* are used to improve the irregular surface of a scar but are not considered for pitted or 'ice pick' acne scars which extend into the deeper layers of the skin. Although done under anaesthetic, this is not a particularly pleasant procedure. A rotating wire brush or a carbon dioxide laser may be used to 'plane' the skin, removing some skin layers. It is like grazing your skin deliberately. It can take several months before the skin (which looks as though you have been sunburned) is regenerated, and you'll need to protect your skin from the sun in the future. Dark or sallow skins are more at risk of getting patchy discolouration than fair skins.

Wrinkles   Fine fair skin which has numerous fine wrinkles because of a lifetime of sun damage is about the only type which should even consider a *chemical face peel*, but because this is an unpleasant and painful procedure, which can cause patchy pigmentation, possible large pores and after which sunbathing should be taboo, it is not something to be undertaken lightly.

Your face is chemically peeled with a phenol preparation, which creates a burn. The tissue around the eyes and mouth may swell dramatically and you may find it hard to see, eat or speak. Your skin ends up looking as though you have had a severe sunburn and will be very sensitive.

Collagen injections   are a form of protein 'Polyfilla' which can fill out wrinkles temporarily – the results last from about six to nine months. The injections may take only about 10 minutes, can sting initially, until the local anaesthetic incorporated into the collagen starts to work, and may leave a slight redness which soon dies away.

They can soften nose-to-mouth lines, frown lines between the brows, forehead lines, crows feet at the outer corners of the eyes (but not too close) and the small lines round the mouth into which lipstick 'bleeds'. They are effective but expensive because of the topping-up needed.

TO MAKE YOU LOOK YOUNGER

Face-lift (rhytidectomy)

This is essentially a neck lift because it gets rid of jowls and double chins, aiming to give a smooth, clean jawline. The optimum time for surgery is between the ages of 45 and 65, and the surgeon's ideal patient is a slim woman in her late 40s or early 50s who wants to look better for her own sake and who fully realizes the limitations of the operation. A full fat face is difficult to treat successfully.

Face-lifts today are more than just skin tightening. The key part is the treatment of the thin sheet of muscle called the platysma, suspended from the jaw and extending into the neck. It is a kind of built-in chin strap. As the muscle ages and loses its tone and gravity takes it toll, the flesh is pulled out of shape, making a bulge in the form of jowls.

The modern face-lift is called a Smas Lift with a 'through and through' dissection. The platysma muscle is tightened to provide better support, the undermined skin in trimmed and lifted and liposuction is used to remove fat from under the chin.

This is a long and major cosmetic operation and you are not going to feel too good for a while, so expect not less than two weeks off work. There is bruising and swelling and possible numbness. The particular nerve that surgeons try to miss lies under the platysma muscle in front of the ear. Dissecting the muscle and pulling on it flirts with danger as there could be possible damage to the nerves of sensation or even worse, motor damage. The motor nerves drive the muscles of the face, and if things go wrong, it could result in a droopy corner to the mouth or an unequal smile. These complications are serious but rare, happily.

About 5 per cent of patients are left with impaired sensation in some area of the face, perhaps around the ears, but it doesn't seem to worry them much.

Eyelid reduction (blepharoplasty)

As the skin ages, we may get loose skin folds on the upper eyelid, or fat can accumulate underneath the eyes, causing bags. Cosmetic eye operations aim to remove excess skin and perhaps lift the muscle under the eye, to make you look younger and less tired.

THE AGEING FACE

THE AGELESS FACE

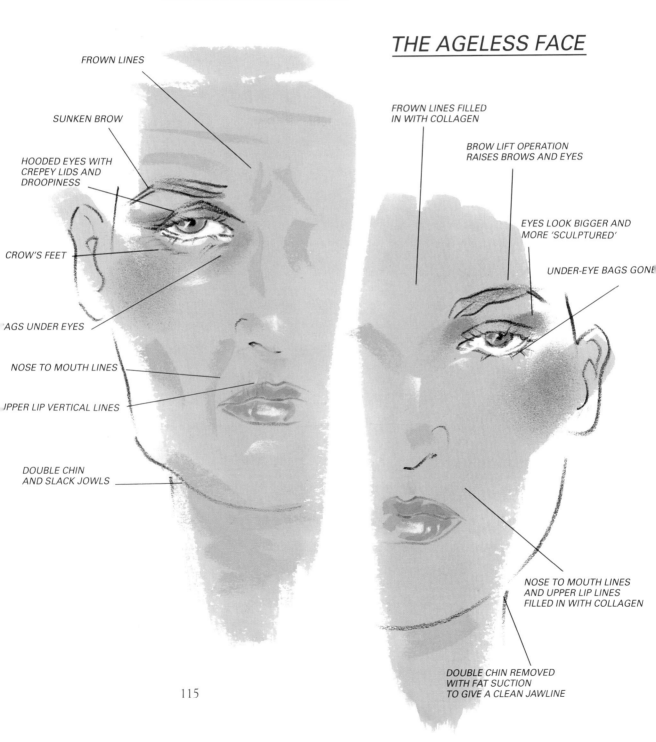

FROWN LINES

SUNKEN BROW

HOODED EYES WITH
CREPEY LIDS AND
DROOPINESS

CROW'S FEET

AGS UNDER EYES

NOSE TO MOUTH LINES

JPPER LIP VERTICAL LINES

DOUBLE CHIN
AND SLACK JOWLS

FROWN LINES FILLED
IN WITH COLLAGEN

BROW LIFT OPERATION
RAISES BROWS AND EYES

EYES LOOK BIGGER AND
MORE 'SCULPTURED'

UNDER-EYE BAGS GONE

NOSE TO MOUTH LINES
AND UPPER LIP LINES
FILLED IN WITH COLLAGEN

DOUBLE CHIN REMOVED
WITH FAT SUCTION
TO GIVE A CLEAN JAWLINE

The upper eyelid reduction operation is relatively quick and trouble-free, given a good surgeon, with the excess skin being cut away and the wound closed with fine sutures in the crease of the eye. Because the skin is extremely thin and delicate, the resulting scar is usually one of the finest possible; it lies within a normal skin fold and ends in the natural creases at the outer corners of the eye, so is hopefully imperceptible.

Surgeons often use local anaesthetics and intravenous sedation rather than a full anaesthetic, for a 'day case' operation. Afterwards, your eyes will be covered with pads for some hours, and there will probably be some bruising and perhaps swelling. You might feel a tightness in the lids and some eye grittiness for a couple of weeks after surgery, but this soon goes.

If too much fat, skin or muscle is removed, then one complication that can occur is pronounced asymmetry of the eyelids – one looking different from the other. Minor adjustments can be made under local anaesthetic to get the right balance.

Reduction of the lower eyelid is a more exacting cosmetic operation, with a cut being made just below the roots of the eyelashes extending outwards into the crowsfeet. The skin is pulled downwards to expose muscle and fat, which are trimmed as necessary. Initially, the scars appear as small red marks at the sides of the eyes, but these fade away.

An unlucky complication would be to get a downward pull on the lower lid, exposing the white of the eye (scleral show) or revealing the red lining of the lid. This is due to too much skin having been removed, perhaps, or bad wound healing.

The brow lift

This operation reduces horizontal and vertical frown lines and lifts the brow, which has sunk with ageing. It may be done at the same time as eyelid reduction.

A big cut is made from ear to ear across the top of the head, with the scar concealed in the hair. Small muscles at the top of the nose and between the brows, which are responsible for vertical frown lines, may be excised together with a horizontal strip of forehead-wrinkling muscle. Skin is pulled up and tightened, and surplus skin trimmed.

You get numbness on the scalp, and perhaps between the brows, for a while. You will get a higher brow, naturally. Some hair may fall out near the cut, but it is well disguised and usually grows again within the year.

FACIAL CORRECTIONS

A new nose (rhinoplasty)

Leonardo da Vinci was convinced that it was the nose above all else that established the psychological character of the face. If Cleopatra had had a different nose, according to legend, the whole face of the earth would have been changed.

Meryl Streep, Barbra Streisand and Sophia Loren may have kept their strong and characteristic noses untouched by cosmetic surgery, but others elect to have surgery to change a nose they find unendurable, and even the removal of a minor bump may make a difference to self confidence.

One of the most popular cosmetic surgery operations, it changes the shape of the nose by altering the underlying bone and cartilage either by removing, altering or adding and then redraping the skin over the new foundations. The operation is performed from inside the nose leaving no external scars.

A surgeon will prefer you to tell him exactly what you do not like about your nose and he will tell you that there are several factors outside his control and skills: the thickness of your skin, for one. A thicker skin is more difficult to drape. The way you heal – we all heal differently – is an unknown quantity, and he will probably advise you that drastic changes are not usually reasonable on both practical and psychological grounds.

Operations on the nose are not painful, but there will be some discomfort. You will have a general anaesthetic and afterwards, your nose will be blocked with packing and you will have to breath through your mouth until it is removed. The swelling and bruising round the eyes settles within a week or two, but the healing process takes at least a further six months.

Chin augmentation

This is sometimes suggested by a surgeon at the same time as a rhinoplasty in order to balance the profile. Or you may seek it if you have a small or receding chin. A silicone implant is inserted through an incision inside the mouth (invisibly) or in the skin of the upper neck (which may leave a small scar). This is usually a successful procedure, and if the implant shifts, giving you a crooked jaw, it can be repositioned.

BODY IMPROVING

Breast uplift (mastoplexy)

Breasts may get slacker and droop after pregnancy and breast-feeding, because of loss of weight, or just because of the effects of gravity and ageing.

This operation aims to tighten the 'envelope' of the breast, removing excess skin and restoring a more attractive cone shape, but leaving the breast volume unchanged. Nothing can remove stretch-marks, although some may be lost when some skin is excised. If you want breast implants as well, you'll need to have two operations about six months apart.

The nipple will be moved, but as it is not detached from the underlying structure, sensitivity should not be too impaired. There will be some scars, but these fade with time, to a certain extent.

Breast augmentation (mamoplasty)

A very popular operation sought by those with naturally small breasts or whose breasts have shrunk following pregnancy, but not without its problems.

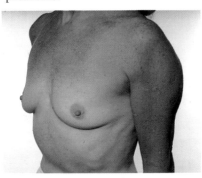

Silicone gel implants are inserted through an incision in the armpit, or just above the crease in the lower part of the breast. There will be some discomfort after surgery, and you'll need to wear a dressing across the top of the chest to hold the implants down, for about two weeks.

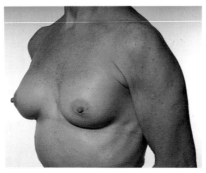

Having new full breasts where once you were flat can be highly satisfactory but possible complications (and up to 50 per cent of patients may get them) can be a fibrous encapsulation, a gradual accumulation of fibrous tissue around the implants, which are after all foreign bodies.

The breasts become firm, losing natural mobility and can become as hard as cricket balls, with the encircling scar perhaps causing distortion. How your body heals or takes the implants is very individual. Surgeons use different techniques to try and avoid capsules with varying success. Some use a polyurethane-covered implant into which the breast tissue grows and this may avoid the worst effects of encapsulation. But should there be an infection, they are difficult to remove.

Treatment for the capsule involves 'breast popping' with the surgeon using powerful squeezing to split the capsule, allowing the breasts to soften and lie naturally. But the capsule often returns. Most breast augmentations have capsule formation, more or less, but if it isn't too bad, most women would find it acceptable. Though the small scars involved usually fade, some patients (those with fair skins and red hair are most at risk) may be unlucky enough to get a thick red raised scar.

One cosmetic surgery operation may not be the end of the story with breast augmentation. So always make sure you talk things through with your surgeon. There may be more fees for other operations.

Breast reduction

Large pendulous breasts can be both an embarrassment and a source of pain and discomfort, with bra straps biting into shoulders, backache, round shoulders, and heat rashes.

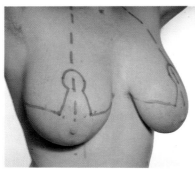

This is a long, major operation, with the surgeon practically dismantling the breasts, shifting the nipples and areola to a higher position, and removing excess breast tissue and skin.

The resulting scarring is considerable, and there is bound to be a loss of nipple sensation – at the worst, a nipple may be lost when the blood supply to it is disturbed, but the surgeon can reconstruct it.

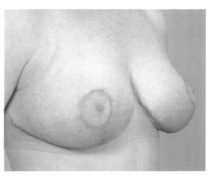

Despite this, women who have this operation are usually happy and satisfied – the trade-off seems worth it to them, as scars may be better than discomfort and embarrassment.

Tummy tuck

Skin that is lax and inelastic, stretched beyond redemption because of pregnancies or having lost a lot of weight, can be smoothed with an abdominal reduction, and liposuction may also be used to remove fatty bulges. But your surgeon will not want to operate if you are still very overweight or intend to become pregnant again.

A low horizontal incision is made in the bikini line, the navel is repositioned, excess skin and fat removed, and a pot belly is flattened by tightening the abdominal muscles with thick permanent sutures.

This is a major operation, and because the abdomen tends not to heal well, you may find a second operation is necessary to tidy up the scars.

After surgery, you'll feel uncomfortable, and you might find the stitches pulling for a while. Expect to wear a tight bandage to support your abdomen, and allow three weeks off work and at least six weeks not doing anything vigorous. There will be swelling and numbness, as well as scarring, but this fades (hopefully). At worst, you might lose your navel, but the surgeon can create a new one successfully.

Fat suction

One of the newest cosmetic techniques, it is increasingly popular to remove fatty bulges on thighs, buttocks, and other parts of the body, and may be used in combination with another operation (such as a face-lift or tummy tuck).

A cannula, connected to a vacuum pump, is inserted into the fat area via a 1 cm incision made in the skin, and fat is sucked out. The area will be firmly bandaged to reduce swelling and bruising, but expect discomfort – like being kicked by a horse. You could experience a most uncomfortable two weeks, but massage and physiotherapy may help bruising to go more quickly. Best on skin which has a good tone so it 'pings' back when the fat is removed. If too much fat is removed, you could get shelving or dents.

CHAPTER 12

BEAT THE CLOCK...

Exercise is one of the best antidotes to ageing. You become stronger, more flexible – stiffness makes you look older. You improve your circulation, your cardiovascular system, your posture and your bones (helping to avoid osteoporosis, the brittle bone disease); it also helps to keep your mind alert.

Join a class – there are so many to chose from these days that you should be able to find one you like. It doesn't have to be aerobics if you can't stand the pounding; there are levels of strenuousness. Low-impact aerobics, for instance, is kinder, or you can do jazz-dancing, yoga, or stretching. If you have a back problem seek out a teacher who is properly trained and who understands and can supervise the right kind of exercises for you.

Join a gym and you can do weight training as well as using exercise bikes, rowers and tread mills. A strong, well-trained body is a young body and makes you feel in control of yourself and your life and being more active actually seems to give you more energy.

Build in challenges. Those who claim to feel mentally younger often tend to enjoy novelty and challenge in their lives. Have you thought about taking up something new – badminton or tennis, joining a swimming club, going cross-country walks, learning T'ai Chi?

And remember, challenges don't all have to be physical. It is mental stimulation that can really make a difference to your attitude to age. If you don't want to lose it, use it, is a maxim we could all follow. Use your brain to keep alert and stimulated – there's always something new to learn, to discover, to experience. If you don't already, do read newspapers to keep up to date with what is going on in the world, and books for inspiration and stimulation.

Don't smoke. Cigarette smoke decreases the amount of oxygen reaching your skin and there is no doubt that it hinders healing. A smoker is going to look older no matter what else she does, and you owe it to your health and your future to give up the weed, however much effort it costs you, because smoking can shorten your life.

121

Eat healthily. Food is your body's fuel and if you don't put in the right octane, you won't get the mileage. You'll feel and look better if you eat nutritiously. That means low-fat, high-fibre, lots of fresh vegetables and fruit, and don't overdo the alcohol.

Slim tips

Being overweight makes you look older than your years, it's a fact . . . an unfortunate fact, if you have spent a lifetime trying to slim and not succeeding. So what are you going to do about it?

Cut down on fat. Latest slimming research seems to indicate that the fat we eat is the fat we wear! Comparatively little energy is used up in digesting fat and it has a natural affinity to the fat in the body: it is just a step away from your mouth to your hips . . . Carbohydrates, on the other hand, such as bread, potatoes, rice and pasta, fruit and vegetables, have a much more complex digestive process and use up more energy before being broken down. So it pays to cut down on fatty meats, frying, the hidden fat in cakes, biscuits and puddings, high fat cheeses and whole milk, and switch to lower fat versions such as skimmed milk.

Take a close look at your lifestyle and see if you can make some long-term changes in what you eat. Crash diets just don't work, because you inevitably put back any weight you have lost when you return to whatever lifestyle made you fat in the first place.

Join a club. Slimming clubs give you group support and motivation and a friendly atmosphere in which to discuss your diet problems. If you have never tried this method of slimming before, it is well worth considering.

Be more active. What you eat is only half the solution. You got fat because you took in more energy than you expended. If you take more exercise, you help the pounds to shift and also make yourself fitter and healthier. Start today with a walk – a brisk walk that makes you feel hot. A gentle stroll is not going to use up much energy.

Get off the bus a stop or two earlier and walk home. Walk up the stairs at work instead of taking the lift. Go for walks in the country at the weekend. Invest in some comfortable light walking boots.

Don't use food as compensation. Food is for eating when you feel hungry, not because you are unhappy. Try to get other compensations. If

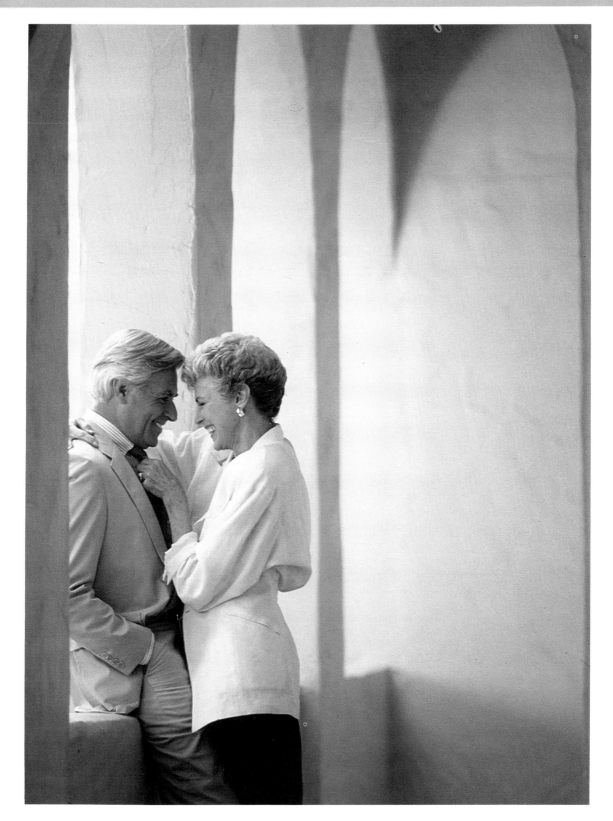

you cannot resist temptations such as chocolate and crisps, don't keep them in the house. You cannot eat what isn't there.

Don't eat on the run. You always tend to eat more when you are not really concentrating – such as when you are watching television. Whenever you have a meal, even a snack, set the table, sit down and do it properly. Take your time – the quicker you eat, the more you'll want.

Substitute. Change from ordinary full-fat milk to skimmed or semiskimmed milk. Try lower-fat hard and soft cheeses, yoghurt or fromage frais instead of cream, sweeteners rather than sugar.

Fill up with vegetables. Fresh fruit and vegetables give you vitamins and fibre and help you to feel fuller. Have a bowl of crudités (raw carrot, cauliflower florets, pieces of pepper, mushrooms etc.) in the fridge ready for dipping into. Make a low-calorie dip with yoghurt, herbs, garlic or onion, Worcestershire or soya sauce.

Eat fresh fruit rather than a sticky desert. Instead of a cream bun, use the money to buy some delicious tropical fruit such as a mango.

Have a bowl of soup – home-made vegetable soup – before each meal, then you will want to eat less. You can make your own vegetable soup, without fat, with all kinds of different vegetables and liquidize it for a smooth and creamy texture.

A question of balance

Always think of yourself as a whole – with beauty and fashion all part of your total look. Check your appearance before you go out in a full-length mirror, and be honest with yourself. Don't fool yourself with wishful thinking but face the facts.

If you are short, take care not to have your hair too 'big' and voluminous, or it may have the effect of making you seem even shorter. A well-cut shorter style may be more flattering.

If you are tall, a close-to-the-head minimalist short cut can make your head seem too small in proportion to the rest of you, and fuller chin or shoulder-length styles will be better.

As you get older very severe hair styles are not all that flattering; it's more softening to have some fullness and movement round the face, though have hair cut to no more than shoulder length, if you prefer it longer. Your style should be determined by your face shape – a good stylist can make all the difference. Aim to find one you can trust and have your style adjusted every few years.

A short neck   can seem longer with hair worn in a swept-up style, off the shoulders; shirt necks with the top buttons undone, V-necks and lower collars, have the same effect, whereas polo necks seem to shorten it even more, and a choker necklace is not in your interest.

A long neck   is to be envied, but if yours is too much of a good thing, you can disguise it with polo necks, scarves and high necked dresses and blouses. Anything too revealing can show a bony neck and shoulders, so covered-up is best.

Upper arms   that are no longer slim and firm should be covered with sleeves or scarves; avoid any sleeveless fashion.

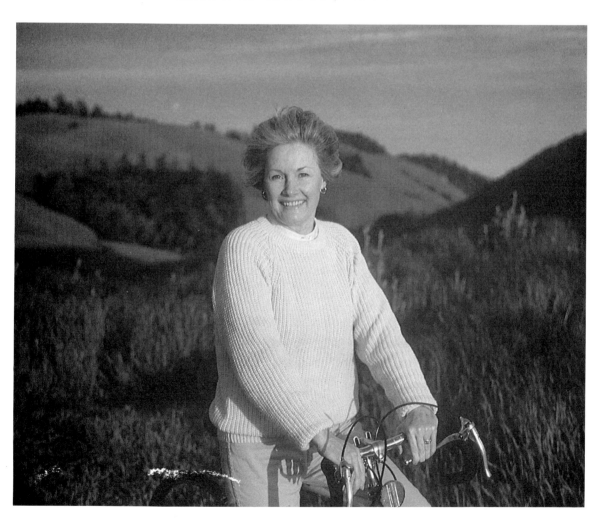

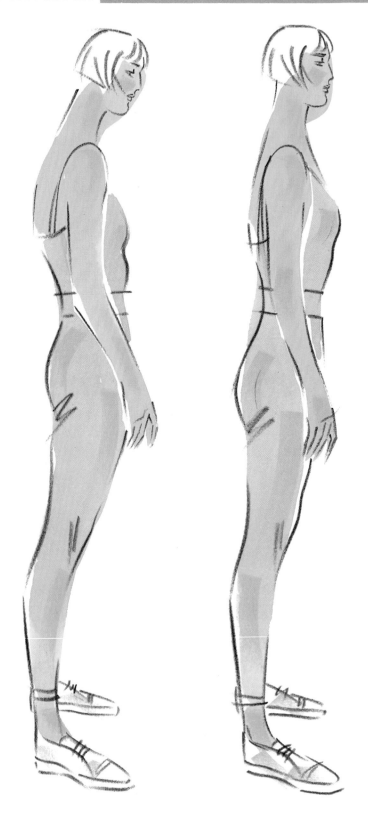

Posture

Posture can make a real difference to how the world perceives you. If you walk around bunched up with bent shoulders, your head poked forward and stomach bulging out, you will seem much older than your years. Actors know that the key to making a performance look older is in how the character walks, stands and sits.

Bad posture   throws the body out of alignment and puts extra strain on the spine, making the neck tilt at an awkward angle so the muscles become stiff and tense. Muscles are fixed to the head both at the base of the skull and at the jawline and run down to be inserted at various points in the back as shoulders. Aches and pains are often caused by holding the shoulders incorrectly. Try rotating each shoulder in turn to remind yourself not to hold them hunched up but comfortably down. If you hold your neck in a set and rigid manner, it can lead to strained neck and muscles and tension headaches.

Good posture   is attractive and gives an impression of youthfulness and energy. When you stand and walk, keep your shoulders back and down but not military stiff. Pull in your stomach and tuck your bottom under. Hold your head high as though you had rope attaching the crown of your head to the ceiling. Stand with feet slightly apart and your weight evenly balanced.

As you hold your shoulders down and relaxed, your neck will lengthen naturally. Never poke your head forward when you sit or walk.

When you sit, make sure you sit right back into the chair, rather than perching on the edge, and have your weight evenly distributed on both buttocks. Have your thighs parallel and comfortable, but not straddled too far apart. Lift your ribcage away from your hips. Do not slump – that always makes you older – but sit upright. If you suffer from varicose veins, remember crossing your legs is bad for the circulation. Your bed should give support to your spine and body so it should be firm. A soft, sagging mattress can give you neck and backache.

Protect your back because the spine is one of the areas of the body most susceptable to stress and injury, and a troublesome back is not only painful but can make you stooped and older than your years. Try not to bend from the lower back when picking up something, but bend your knees. You should not have to curve your spine to read or do office work – a good, back-supporting chair is of great importance.

INDEX OF BEAUTY PROBLEMS

acne	16, 19
acne scars	113
ageing hands	72
alopecia	99-100
athlete's foot	80
birthmarks	112
blisters	81
blushing	69, 70
brittle nails	73
breasts, too large	119
breasts, too small	118
bunions	80
chilblains	81
corns and calluses	80
contact lenses	56-7
cramps	81
crêpey neck	88
double chin	71
eye bags	70
eyes, too close together	55
eyebrows, too thick	52
eyebrows, too thin	53
fine hair	97-8
fragile nails	73
full face	71
greying hair	100-105
hair, dry	93-4
hair loss	99-100
hard skin	80
heat rash	54
ingrown toe-nails	80
lipstick bleeding, feathering	61
lipstick changing colour	60
lips, one fuller than the other	63
lips, thin	62
lips, too full	62
lips, turning downwards	63
long neck	125
moles	112
mouth too wide	63
nail biting	73
narrow face	71
neck wrinkles	88
oily skin	21, 22, 25
older eyes	55
over-processed hair	92, 96
port wine stains	112
prickly heat	33
prominent eyes	54
prominent nose	70, 117
sensitive skin	25
short neck	125
skin allergy	23, 33, 72
skin cancer	19-20, 31
skin dehydration	10, 12
skin tanning	27, 33
slimming	122, 124
small eyes	54
smelly feet	81
split ends	93
spots	14-16
tattoos	113
veruccas	81
wrinkles	69, 112

USEFUL ADDRESSES

Weight Watchers (UK) Ltd
Sovereign House
229 Oxford Street
London W1 1LA
071 491 1929

Keep-Fit Association
16 Upper Woburn Place
London WC1H 0QG
071 387 4349

The British Association of Aesthetic Plastic Surgeons (BAAPS)
The Royal College of Surgeons
35-43 Lincoln's Inn Fields
London WC2A 3PN
071 636 4864

Women's Health Concern
83 Earls Court Road
London W8 6AU
071 938 3932

Federation of Image Consultants
Mallory House
27 Verulam Road
St Albans
Herts AL3 4DG
0727 44682

Joan Price's Face Place
33 Cadogan Street
London SW3 2PP
071 589 9062

Stephen Glass at Face Facts
73 Wigmore Street
London W1H 9LH
071 486 8287

Richard Dalton at Claridges
Claridges Hotel
Brook Street
London W1A 2JQ
071 409 1517

FURTHER READING

Lizzie Webb's Total Health and Fitness (Boxtree)
Cosmetic Surgery: A Consumer Guide by Denise Winn (Optima)
A Woman In Your Own Right by Anne Dickson (Pan)

PICTURE CREDITS

p.11: L'Oréal's Plénitude skincare range includes Aqua Cleansing Cream, a rinsable cream cleanser, that is not as dehydrating as soap.

p.13: Lancôme's Noctosome system is based on time-release microspheres, encapuslating skincare ingredients.

p.15: Clarins plant treatment range for oily/combination skins includes Gentle Foaming Cleanser, Toning Lotion, and Lotus treatment cream.

p.18: The 2000 range of skincare and colour cosmetics from Boots includes a 2000 Localised Wrinkle Treatment.

p.23: Boots 2000 Treatment Facial Wash.

p.26: Conquête du Soleil suncare range with natural plant extracts combines ultra violet protection with skincare.

p.28: Uvistat's Lipscreen protects from sun and wind, helps to prevent cracking and inflammation.

p.30/31: Revlon Sun is a comprehensive range of water-resistant sunscreen products designed to prepare, protect and prolong a tan.

p.32: Uvistat's range of broad spectrum sun protection products have skin protecting filters as well as screening against burning UVB.

pp.35, 38-9: Lancôme's Blush Majeur combines the qualities of both a cream and a powder blusher, can be applied with fingers (for a natural look) or a brush (for a more sculptured effect). Build up colour gradually, layer upon layer.

p.43: Christian Dior's 5 colour eyeshadow palette 'Mist' includes dark brown, ecru, matt black, smoke grey and cloudy violet; everything you need for shading, sculpting, highlighting and lining.

p.43: Lancôme's L'Origine range of eye

make-up: Duo Jeux d'Ombres powder shadow in Gris Pierre contains a pastel grey enlivened with sunflower yellow. Eyes are emphasised with Traceur Matic liquid eyeliner close to lashes in Gris Argent shade.

p.44: Sensiq cosmetics and skincare are fragrance-free and screened for irritants. The eye make-up range includes crease-resistant powder eye colour and a fine felt-tipped eyeliner pen.

p.46: L'Oréal's Plénitude skincare range includes oil-free Active Daily Moisture lotion, for combination skins or for summer when you want something light.

p.47: Lancôme's eyeshadow duo Jeux d'Ombres comes in a browny-pink combination called Bois de Cedre.

p.48: Rimmel's wide range of eye cosmetics includes soft, easy-to-apply eye pencils and long-lasting mascaras.

p.51: Helena Rubinstein Volumatic mascara incorporates a treatment cream formula and bio-protein ingredients for holding power.

p.58: Elizabeth Arden Lip-Fix Creme, a pre-lipstick treatment, stops colour 'bleeding' into the tiny lines around the mouth. The Luxury Lipstick range has a moist formulation that also resists feathering and fading.

p.61: Boots No. 7 lipsticks provide both colour and moisture.

pp.74-5: Sally Hansen's wide range of nail treatments include a nail strengthener (a protective shield applied under and over nail varnish), and a nail smoother (to fill in ridges prior to applying nail colour).

p.75: Chanel products cover everything you need for a manicure – from cuticle softener and nail strengthening oil to protective base coat and top coat.

p.79: Scholl has a wide range of products for pedicure and foot problems.

p.87: Sophisticated 'dressed' style by Richard Dalton of Claridges, for Clairol. Longer hair is swept up and back into a French pleat, keeping height on the crown. Freeze Forming Spray from Clairol Professional range gives lasting hold.

p.89: Helena Rubinstein Intercell cream helps skin hydration, smoothes roughness.

p.90: Immaculately dressed hair for evening by Richard Dalton of Claridges, for Clairol. Eminence perm for tinted hair gives body, and the hair has also been coloured with Clairol Plus salon treatment colour in True Golden Blonde. Freeze Forming Spray helps keep the style in place.

p.95: BaByliss Professional range of electrical hair appliances includes a cordless heat styling brush which controls unruly curly hair or adds body and volume to straight hair.

p.96: Volume and waves for shorter hair using Clairol's Take Two heated tongs.

p.98: L'Oréal Studio Line Sculpting Mousse gives lasting body and hold and adds volumes to curls and waves.

p.98: Elida Gibbs' Dimension 2-in-1 conditioning shampoo gives one-step care and stops static. There are variants for normal hair/frequent use, dry/treated hair and dandruff control.

p.101: Grey hair is enhanced with Clairol's Loving Care semi-permanent colourant in Silver Slate. An effective after-colour leave-in conditioner is included in the pack.

p.102: Clairol's Loving Care semi-permanent in Silver Slate is used to condition grey hair and reduce the tendency to yellowing.

p.103: Make-up artist Celia Hunter's magnificent white hair has always been one of her most distinctive features. Clairol's Loving Care semi-permanent in Silver Pearl gives subtle enhancement.

p.105: If you don't want to go grey, home hair colourants are easy to use. Clairesse gentle permanent hair colour in Light Ash Blonde gives subtle tones.

p.106: Revlon's Flex Balsam and Protein body building shampoo and conditioner for extra body, while the Flex Body Building Styling Mousse adds control for crisper styling.

p.107: RoC's Cream eyeshadow in Sable is used as a base, with fine powder shadow in Brun Soleil blended on top. Sheer Lip Balm moisturizes lips and provides a hint of a tint.

pp.6, 65-8 and jacket: Hair by Richard Dalton at Claridges. Brushes from Stephen Glass at Face Facts). Photography by Peter Underwood. Make-up artist Vanessa Haines.

Make-up by Max Factor mainly from the Swedish Formula, fragrance-free, hypo-allergenic cosmetics collection.

Face: Max Factor Erace concealer in fair, Swedish Forumla Liquid Foundation in ivory, loose Finishing Powder in translucent matte. Powder Blusher in rosebud.

Eyes: Swedish Formula Duo in Moonbeam, and Sienna Silks (which was also used on eyebrows) and Max Factor Eyeshadow Duos in Golden Coral and Silver Leaf. Swedish Formula mascara in brownish black specially formulated for sensitive eyes.

Lipstick: Swedish Formula Damson Dusk.